ASSESSING
INTERVENTIONS

RESEARCH METHODS FOR PRIMARY CARE

Series Board of Editors

The goal of RESEARCH METHODS FOR PRIMARY CARE is to address important topics meeting the needs of the growing number of primary care researchers. Purposely following a sequence from general principles to specific techniques, implementation strategies, and dissemination, the series volumes each examine a particular aspect of primary care research, emphasizing actually conducting research in the real world. The well-known contributors bring an international, multidisciplinary perspective to the volumes, enhancing their usefulness to primary care researchers.

Volumes in the series:

ASSESSING INTERVENTIONS

TRADITIONAL AND INNOVATIVE METHODS

EDITED BY

FRED TUDIVER
MARTIN J. BASS
EARL V. DUNN
PETER G. NORTON
MOIRA STEWART

**Research Methods
for Primary Care**
Volume 4

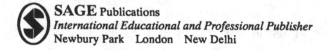

SAGE Publications
International Educational and Professional Publisher
Newbury Park   London   New Delhi

For information address:

SAGE Publications, Inc.
2455 Teller Road
Newbury Park, California 91320

SAGE Publications Ltd.
6 Bonhill Street
London EC2A 4PU
United Kingdom

SAGE Publications India Pvt. Ltd.
M-32 Market
Greater Kailash I
New Delhi 110 048 India

Printed in the United States of America

Library of Congress Cataloging-in-Publication Data

Main entry under title:

Assessing interventions / edited by Fred Tudiver . . . [et al.].
    p. cm. — (Research methods for primary care ; v. 4)
    Includes bibliographical references and index.
    ISBN 0-8039-4770-4. — ISBN 0-8039-4771-2 (pbk.)
    1. Clinical trials. 2. Family medicine—Research—Methodology.
3. Medical care—Evaluation. I. Tudiver, Fred. II. Series.
R853.C55A77   1992
362.1′068′5—dc20   92-19922

94 95 10 9 8 7 6 5 4 3 2

Sage Production Editor: Diane S. Foster

Contents

Foreword: Assessing Interventions in Primary Care

BRIAN K. HENNEN

"The profession of medicine, as part of its own culture, has built
some safeguards against the abuse of the sense of omnipotence. I
know of no other structured area of human activity in which open
self-criticism is so much a part."

Eric Cassell

This book is about self-criticism in primary care practice through
research, about how primary care clinicians intervene in the lives
of the people they serve. Assessing interventions in primary care
is essential to improve practice. Most health professionals have
been taught to avoid doing harm while trying to do good. But when
only about one third of today's medical interventions have been
found by modern scientific methods to be of established benefit,
one third are of uncertain benefit and one third are suspect of not
being beneficial at all, such surveillance is long overdue.

We must assess our own interventions in primary care. But when
new technology and new pharmacology are developed and initiated in tertiary care settings, our task in primary care is made more
complex because we must also assess these interventions. Applied
frequently by our subspecialty colleagues in more controlled and
tidy institutional settings to a very ill subset of patients, such
interventions are sometimes mistakenly assumed to be appropriate
for direct transfer to a more heterogeneous group of patients in the
relatively uncontrolled and messy ambulatory community setting.

The assessment task is enormous and can only reasonably be tackled by preparing all primary care health professionals to be curious, critical, and forever vigilant about interventions applied to individuals in their practices.

Further, we are supported by increasing evidence in our belief that a patient-centered approach is how primary care should be provided. In patient-centered caring, patient-doctor relationships or client-professional relationships are fundamental. Research of these relationships is difficult, as Korsch (1989) points out, but parallel with adverse drug reactions, much harm can be done when relationships between client and therapist go astray. Balint's doctor drug can have undesirable side effects (1972). Personal professional interventions deserve assessment for their efficacy with equivalent rigor as do technological or pharmaceutical ones. We need a broader view of the task.

This leads directly to the application of suitable methods of assessment—quantitative and qualitative—bean counting and tasting the coffee, and in the qualitative we are now moving forward. To indicate the validity of qualitative assessment, I counter comments about "hard" and "soft" data with the reminder that multitest biochemical screens of healthy individuals have a substantial likelihood of showing one or more abnormal results. I argue that such tests are less important than the ability of competent family physicians to identify previously unrecognized depression in their practice population. The lab tests with their numbers are called *hard*. The diagnostic acumen of the family physicians is called *soft*. A second example stems from work by Carol McWilliam (in press) in which detailed qualitative assessments are described of the determinants of hospital admission and discharge decisions. They show that personal concerns of patients, their families, and the many health professionals involved in their care are at least as important in predicting outcomes as diagnostic codes and management resource estimates. But the latter are used almost exclusively by hospital planners. With acceptance of qualitative methodologies as legitimate assessment techniques, our clinical and health care planning decisions will be greatly improved.

If only one third of medical interventions overall have been proven to be effective, then two thirds are in doubt. In primary care most new illness is self-limiting and probably half is never definitively diagnosed. What more important justification for giving greater credibility to studies that report negative findings? In setting out to "prove" (*p* value .05 or less) therapeutive effectiveness, it is as important to show no proven effectiveness. Our journals must report good studies showing negative findings. We must know which of our interventions cannot be "proven" effective.

Iatrogenic illness continues to occur both in and out of hospital. With increased ability to determine potentially harmful drug interactions through computer technology, now available in the smallest solo practice, we can look forward to reducing the frequency of adverse drug interactions. But certain pressures threaten the likelihood of eliminating them altogether. One is the escalating number of new pharmaceutical agents, aggressively promoted by their manufacturers. Another is the self-medicating imperative of society, encouraged inadvertently by the increased empowerment of lay persons to determine the management of their own health care. In the practitioner's office this may translate into an expectation for an antibiotic *now* for the sore throat in spite of the clinician's *wait and see* advice. And the computer can't warn about an interaction if one of the interventions is a self-administered, over-the-counter chemical unknown to the practitioner and not keyed into the computer terminal.

With interventions that are proven effective, we anticipate some risk of doing harm. The balance between potential benefit and risk has to be assessed in every situation. That is when clinical judgment and discussion with an informed patient results in a mutual management decision. When interventions that are not proven effective result in harm, we have the worst cases.

All of these health-seeking behaviors are susceptible to research and should be part of our intervention assessments. How the patient intervenes in illness is at least as important as what we do as health care professionals.

This book compiles the advice of experienced primary care researchers. They are showing us how we can better evaluate our professional behavior. Thank goodness it is they, primary care colleagues, who have undertaken this work! They know the variable nature of our practices. They appreciate our context and our working conditions. Their work is relevant and timely. We owe it to our patients to follow their direction in assessing interventions and we owe it to our students to teach them how.

References

Balint, M. (1972). *The doctor, his patient, and the illness* (p.229). New York: International Universities Press.

Cassell, E. J. (1989). *The healer's art.* Cambridge: MIT Press.

Korsch, B. M. (1989). The past and the future of research in doctor-patient relations. In M. Stewart & D. Roter (Eds.). *Communicating with medical patients* (pp. 246-251). Newbury Park, CA: Sage.

McWilliam, C. (In press). From hospital to home: The elderly's discharge experience. *Family Medicine.*

Acknowledgments

The editors would like to thank the Physicians' Services Incorporated Foundation, Ontario for their generous support for the production of this volume. They also thank the Ontario Ministry of Health and the National Health Research and Development Program (NHRDP) of the Federal Government of Canada for financial support. Anne Stilman helped with the preparation of the manuscript. Without the tireless efforts of Jamie Jensen, this volume would not exist. Thank you all.

Introduction

This book is a natural follow-up to the three previous volumes of this series, which have taken us from asking questions, to using the tools, to the cutting edge of qualitative methods. Here we examine how to best use the results of these investigations when we intervene with our patients, by learning and using scientifically sound methods to evaluate these interventions.

This book is about research methods that can be used successfully to assess interventions in primary care settings. Although at first glance this topic would appear to be well covered in the epidemiological literature, our experience suggests that the issues relating to primary care, because of its general, broad-based nature, are different and often unique and require adaptation of methodologies that have been developed for other health care fields.

The volume is divided into four parts. The first part considers some basic issues in assessing interventions in primary care. Part II examines two major assessment strategies: quantitative methodologies (the traditional approach) and qualitative methodologies (some of which are new to primary care). Part III explores several specific topics, which are illustrated by practical examples. The single chapter in Part IV presents a panel discussion that outlines possible future directions; one in particular is the challenge for the primary care discipline to define its own foci of research activities.

The contributions here should be useful to both novice and experienced researchers, whether community based or academic, as well as to writers and reviewers of grant applications and scientific papers.

Fred Tudiver

PART I

Interventions
in Primary Care

As this book is about interventions in primary care and how to evaluate them rigorously and scientifically, it is appropriate to begin by examining some basics. The two chapters in this section explore the foundation of such assessments—the therapeutic trial. Dr. Gehlbach, a health educator and expert on critical appraisal, presents several traditional therapeutic trials to illustrate the importance of the use of controls, especially concurrent controls, in their evaluation. In particular, he argues for the importance of the concept of placebo controls, contending that it is only by satisfying this minimal standard that we can validly test the efficacy of our treatments.

Dr. Bain, a professor of primary medical care in the United Kingdom, describes several therapeutic trials he undertook in busy community family practices. He uses the term *trials and tribulations* in his title because of the problems and complexities he discovered along the way—problems that might not have been noticed if the research had been carried out in the usual hospital bed "laboratory" or specialist clinic. His contribution presents a model of research team effort in a community-type practice and highlights the fundamental requirements for successful treatment trials in primary care, including the fact that they must be based on the reality of daily practice.

1 Traditional Interventions in Primary Care: Issues of Control

STEPHEN H. GEHLBACH

Clinicians have been in the business of evaluating therapeutic interventions since the medical profession began. It is in the natural order of things. We need to prove—both to our patients and to ourselves—that our treatments work. Efficacious therapy is the bedrock upon which our practices build and professional pride depends. More to the point, when patients get better, we feel good. But, while the rewards of providing effective care are obvious, the optimal methods for achieving this are more elusive. The path to answering the seemingly straightforward question, "Do our treatments work?" turns with some deceptive bends. We will explore a familiar, well-trod portion of this pathway looking for some examples from the recent and not-so-recent past to guide us to an enlightened course.

Case Reports and Case Series

The following is a report of a novel approach to an important clinical problem: restoring function to paralyzed limbs. The technique involves a type of electrotherapy:

> My method was, to place the patient first in a chair, on an electric stool, and draw a number of large strong sparks from all parts of the affected limb or side. Then I fully charged two six-gallon glass jars, each of which had about three square feet of surface coated; and I sent

3

the united shock of these through the affected limb or limbs, repeating the stroke commonly three times each day. The first thing observed, was an immediate greater sensible warmth in the lame limbs that had received the stroke, than in the others; and the next morning the patients usually related, that they had in the night felt a pricking sensation in the flesh of the paralytic limbs; and would sometimes show a number of small red spots, which they supposed were occasioned by those prickings. The limbs, too, were found more capable of voluntary motion, and seemed to receive strength. A man, for instance, who could not the first day lift the lame hand from off his knee, would the next day raise it four or five inches, the third day higher; and on the fifth day was able, but with a feeble languid motion, to take off his hat. (Cohen, 1941)

This description is rather cursory and may sound dated to some, but it represents a lovely illustration of the oldest traditional form of clinical evaluation: the case report or case series. The physician/evaluator administers a new medication or innovative surgical procedure to the patient/subject; then they both wait and watch for the flaccid limb to move, the pain to subside, or the inflammation to recede. Success! The patient improves and returns to social productivity, and the doctor moves on to the next paralyzed leg, migraine headache, or case of cellulitis. As more successful cases are added to the series, confidence grows that the treatment is, indeed, beneficial.

Occasionally, the practitioner becomes more circumspect. Was it really the electrical impulses that restored activity to the flaccid limb, or is there some other factor that might have contributed to the patient's improvement? In the case of the practitioner whose work is described above, one Benjamin Franklin (1757/1941) of Philadelphia, some alternative explanations are provided. Franklin went on to report (in a letter of 1757 to Dr. John Pringle) that it was possible that the improvement among his patients might have arisen not from the electric shocks he was administering, but from "the exercise in the patients' journey, and coming daily to my house, or from the spirits given by the hope of success, enabling them to exert more strength in moving their limbs."

So, in his report, Franklin, although an amateur in the healing business (lacking proper licensing or specialty board certification), not only illustrates the case study approach to treatment evaluation but also provides a cogent critique that highlights the type of methodological problems that make our task of evaluating interventions so difficult. Is the treatment itself responsible for improvement, or are the patient's expectations creating a self-fulfilling prophecy in which the will to recover is primarily responsible for the salubrious effect?

This well-recognized benefit, known as the placebo effect, has been embedded in the healer-patient relationship since such relationships began thousands of years ago. Both parties have a keen desire to see the problem improve, and the power that the mind can exert over bodily afflictions has been demonstrated repeatedly by some of our most intelligent and articulate numbers. In 1910, the psychologist William James, who knew the human mind as well as anyone of his day, wrote to a confidant, Sir William Osler, about his hopes for remedy from another form of electrotherapy:

> My anginoid pain has increased during the past year, tho' nitroglycerin stops it like magic. I go to Paris to consult one Dr. Montier, whose high frequency currents have performed a *wunder kur* on a neighbor of mine (reducing his arterial tension from 230mm to 150 in four applications) with a relief of all his formidable symptoms, that has now been complete for six months! I know of two cases of similar relief by him, tho' I am unacquainted with the details. It sounds impossible, and I hear that M. is regarded as a quack by medical opinion. Nevertheless, I don't wish to leave that stone unturned, since my own trouble (in which I gladly acknowledge an element of nervous hyperaesthesia) seems progressive. (Edelstein, 1946, p. 292)

More recently, we had the example of Norman Cousins (1976), former editor of the *Saturday Review*, who wrote of his recovery from a mysterious ailment through hefty doses of vitamin C and "belly laughter."

Such benefits of the power of positive thinking notwithstanding, when we are trying to decide whether an expensive pharmacological agent or risky surgical procedure is worthwhile, it is essential to separate the role played by the placebo effect from that of the intervention itself.

Placebos and Expectations

Dr. Henry Beecher (1955) wrote on the magnitude and breadth of the placebo effect in intervention studies, cataloging examples for a host of ailments ranging from postoperative wound pain to the common cold. He found the effect to be not only of substantial magnitude but also remarkably consistent over 14 studies. On average, 35% of more than 1,000 patients evaluated in these studies responded to a placebo medication with a range between 20% and 50%.

Few examples of the placebo effect are as compelling as those in the literature on William James's affliction, angina pectoris. Benson and McCallie (1979) provide a documentary on the mischief the placebo effect has played in evaluating angina remedies, reviewing case-series reports from the 1930s and 1940s on the use of xanthines, khellin, and vitamin E as well as 1950s and 1960s studies of internal mammary artery ligation and implantation. Each of these therapies has subsequently fallen into disuse and disrepute; however, some 13 studies involving more than 1,100 subjects indicated subjective improvements ranging as high as 80%.

Benson and McCallie attribute these remarkable successes not only to the power of the placebo effect but to a "contagious" enthusiasm of the experimenters as well. In one study reported by Dr. George Leroy (1941), aminophylline (a xanthine drug) was tested as an antiangina medication. Sensitive to the fact that there was considerable skepticism over the merits of xanthine prescriptions for the purpose, he added credibility to his case series by including a "suitably controlled series of patients" who received placebo pills. But Leroy himself was well aware of the identity of the compounds he was administering, reporting that "no rigid schedule of courses of active drug and placebo was adhered to." Rather, he adjusted aminophylline dosages until an improvement was apparent. His placebos were "seldom administered for a period longer than two weeks," but the active drug would be given for 4 to 10 weeks. Among 68 patients treated with either aminophylline or placebo, aminophylline was effective 70% to 80% of the time compared with a placebo response of only 17% to 20%. In declaring the success of his trial, Leroy offers a revealing side observation:

In this connection should be mentioned the psychologic attitude of the clinician toward the drugs in question. It is just as unfair in seeking a patient's evaluation of a drug to lead him to expect poor results as to lead him to anticipate good ones. I attempted to be as noncommittal as possible, but discerning patients may well have seen my enthusiasm for these particular xanthine drugs. (p. 924)

The above demonstrates how a case series can suffer from biases introduced by expectant patients and enthusiastic experimenters. The legitimate question arises concerning whether the approach has any role in understanding the value of treatments. It is proposed that case studies can be useful, but their role comes in the formative rather than the summative stages of evaluation. Consider a chapter from early in the story of surgical approaches to angina. In 1951, Drs. Arthur Vineberg and Gavin Miller reported on three patients who underwent internal mammary artery implantation into the left cardiac ventricle in hopes of provoking collateral circulation to anoxic myocardia. Two of the three survived surgery and experienced substantial relief from their pain. In summarizing their experiment, Vineberg and Miller come to several conclusions. First, they state that the internal mammary artery can be successfully implanted into the human heart, with apparently little disturbance to cardiac function. So far so good; they indeed demonstrate the *feasibility* of the operation. But, when they take the next step to claim that the procedure produces relief from angina, it becomes another matter: a matter of separating surgical from placebo effects.

The "Vineberg procedure" became extremely popular; an estimated 10,000 to 15,000 of these operations were performed before it was abandoned (Benson & McCallie, 1979). The evidence that contributed to its fall from grace included several uncontrolled case-series studies. Two reports, published in *Lancet* (Balcon, Leaver, Ross, Ross, & Sowton, 1970) and in the *American Journal of Cardiology* (Langston, Kerth, Selzer, & Cohn, 1972), provided clinical and angiographic follow-up of patients who had undergone the procedure for severe ischemic heart disease. (In neither study was a control group used.) Although subjective reports from patients were extremely encouraging, results of objective assessment painted a different picture. Partial or total relief of angina was reported among 29 of 37 survivors one year following the operation;

angiography, however, demonstrated little physiological basis for this improvement. Only six patients showed substantially improved coronary artery circulation; five of these improved symptomatically. By comparison, an identical proportion (five sixths) of patients with completely occluded implants also said they felt improved. The lack of physiological plausibility created serious doubts as to the true effectiveness of this surgical procedure. The rest, as they say, is history.

Historical Controls

Most experienced researchers and research consumers now expect some comparison population to be included as part of a treatment evaluation. Just who these control patients are, however, and how they are best selected is a subject of debate. Many purists will consider only a concurrently selected, randomly chosen comparison population as adequate. Others have argued a more moderate course: Because full-blown randomized clinical trials can be exceedingly costly and difficult to mount, they are persuaded that another traditional approach, the historical control study, remains a useful alternative (Gehan & Freireich, 1974; Lasagna, 1982).

Table 1.1 illustrates the results of a historical control study. In this experiment, the investigator was attempting to demonstrate the benefits of a new antiseptic system on survival rates for surgical patients undergoing limb amputations. A death rate of approximately 16% from fatal infections or hemorrhagic shock is recorded at the participating hospital following the introduction of the new technique. Before deciding whether this represents an improvement, however, some comparison with the rate that might have been expected had the intervention not been introduced is required. To obtain such an estimate, the author uses a historical control group made up of patients who had had amputations in the two-year period before the introduction of the system. The death rate in those two years was almost 50%. This reduction looks to be a substantial improvement, but several questions come immediately to mind. Were other improvements made to the surgical procedures or hospital care during the time the antiseptic system was initiated? Because most of the deaths occurred from infection, had new antibiotics been added to the medical arsenal? Was the

Table 1.1 Effects of an Antiseptic System on Hospital Mortality

Amputation Site	Number	Deaths
During two years before introduction of the system:		
Shoulder	1	1
Arm	5	3
Forearm	5	1
Thigh	5	4
Knee	8	3
Ankle	5	2
Total	29	14
During three years after introduction of the system		
Shoulder	3	0
Arm	3	0
Forearm	6	1
Thigh	2	1
Knee	13	4
Ankle	9	0
Total	36	6

SOURCE: Adapted from Lister (1870).

severity of cases comparable in the two periods, or did the post-intervention group consist of patients at lower risk?

Such basic questions of method apparently did not concern Joseph Lister when he reported his results of carbolic acid antisepsis in *Lancet* in 1870. And, in fairness, because it would be almost a decade before Koch would launch the bacteriological era, it seems unlikely that a change in the hospital's antibiotic formulary was responsible. History has been kinder to Lister's observations than to Vineberg's: Because we now agree with some unanimity that keeping surgical wounds free of bacterial contamination promotes recovery, we are inclined to be less critical of Lister's potentially flawed study design.

The use of historical controls is, however, fraught with the very kinds of perils that might be imagined from the antisepsis example. Such controls are intended to provide a baseline against which to measure interventions. But, if the subject populations that constitute the baseline and intervention groups differ with respect to severity, comorbid conditions, or other features that may affect outcome, or if events that might exert either a beneficial or a deleterious effect occur between the "control" and intervention periods, the role of the therapy under scrutiny is impossible to assess.

An illustration of the hazards inherent in the historical control comes from an evaluation of cold vaccines (Diehl, Baker, & Cowan, 1938). Study subjects were students at the University of Minnesota who volunteered to participate "because they were particularly susceptible to colds." Recruits gave a history of the number and severity of colds they had experienced during the previous year. They then received subcutaneous, killed vaccine consisting of pneumococci, streptococci, and "bacillus influenzi." During the first year of follow-up, students were instructed to report to the health service whenever a cold developed. They were also required to keep a log, recording each cold they experienced that lasted 24 hours or more.

Among the 272 vaccinated students, the average number of colds tallied during the year following vaccination was 1.6. This compares with the report for the prior year of an average count of 5.9 per subject—a dramatic reduction! It tempts one to abandon parochial thinking about the viral etiology of colds and begin grinding up more bacterial antigens. Several factors have to be considered, however. To begin with, we are comparing counts of upper respiratory infections *documented* through visits to the health service and log books, with students' *recall* of events past. These are not likely to be data of equivalent quality. Memories may overestimate the frequency of previous afflictions or telescope events occurring over many months into a shorter span of time. Second, perhaps the two years under comparison were different with respect to the epidemiology of respiratory infections in the community. Many diseases are cyclical in nature and it may be that the "control" year was particularly laden with epidemics whereas the postintervention year was particularly light. Third, it is possible that the apparent improvement was simply due to a "regression effect." Whenever subjects are selected to participate in an experiment on the basis of some extreme characteristic, such as high blood pressure, low hemoglobin, or propensity to catch cold, there is a statistical tendency for the group as a whole to demonstrate a less extreme average value in subsequent measurements. (See Gehlbach, 1988, for a detailed explanation of this phenomenon.) In this illustration, regression simply means that, if one observes only subjects who had a much higher than average experience with colds last year,

Table 1.2 Status of Tuberculosis 12 Months After Admission

Group (number)	Improvement Number (%)	No Change Number (%)	Deterioration Number (%)	Death Number (%)
Streptomycin (55)	31 (56)	4 (7)	8 (15)	12 (22)
Control (52)	16 (31)	5 (10)	7 (13)	24 (46)

SOURCE: From British Medical Research Council (1948).

they are, as a group, likely to have fewer colds (moved toward the average) the following year, regardless of the concoction injected into their arms.

Fortunately for this example, the investigators included a comparison group of 276 students who were given subcutaneous administrations of saline on the same dosage schedule as those receiving the vaccine. While the vaccinated group showed a 73% reduction in colds from its historical control, the placebo group showed a decline almost as dramatic: 63%.

Some still argue the value of historical controls for study of "diseases that don't go away if untreated or that have predictable courses" (Lasagna, 1982). Such circumstances are rare, and the assumption that one knows just what to expect from a disease in a patient population is risky. In trials of streptomycin as treatment for tuberculosis (British Medical Research Council, 1948), patients were included if they had "acute, progressive, bilateral pulmonary tuberculosis" for which the "estimated chances of spontaneous regression must be small." Although the course for this group of patients seemed predictable, investigators included a concurrent control group of randomly assigned subjects who received no streptomycin.

The results of this study, displayed in Table 1.2, demonstrate the risk of assuming that the prognosis for untreated patients is a foregone conclusion: 31% of subjects in the control group were improved at the time of final evaluation. Not all succumbed to the disease; nor, of course, did all those administered streptomycin survive. The study did provide strong evidence for the effectiveness of streptomycin in treatment of tuberculosis; however, it also shows up the folly of believing that we can be certain of the natural history of a disease.

Volunteer Controls

Having relegated two "tried-and-not-so-true" traditional approaches to evaluation, the case series and the historical control study, to the sidelines, one last type of comparison problem should be considered: the nonrandomly allocated, or "volunteer," control. The solution to the inadequacies of the historical control clearly lies in enlisting comparison subjects who may be observed concurrently with individuals receiving the intervention. This way, the confusion that can result from cyclical variations in severity of epidemics, and simultaneous or competing interventions, is minimized, because the comparison subjects and the experimental subjects should encounter similar historical forces. Even when subjects are selected concurrently, however, problems can occur if they are not chosen such that intervention and comparison groups are composed of similar individuals.

An instructive example again comes from the ischemic heart disease literature. A study reported in the early 1970s (Rechnitzer, Packard, Pavio, Yuhasz, & Cunningham, 1972) tried to evaluate the benefits of exercise for men who had sustained myocardial infarctions. Did a program of exercise rehabilitation lessen the chances of future cardiac death or nonfatal recurrence? Study subjects consisted of 68 male volunteers who had suffered a recent heart attack and subsequently enrolled in the exercise program. Controls were obtained by reviewing medical records to find patients who were hospitalized during the same time as exercise subjects but who did not elect to participate in the exercise program.

Results of this study indicate that exercise is highly effective: The occurrence of cardiac death was reduced by half and that of nonfatal recurrence by almost 75%. But was this control group adequate for the task? Ideally, comparison subjects should provide an estimate of the baseline risk for heart attack survivors who are similar to the exercisers in every respect except participation in the program. But are these groups really similar? Why did comparison subjects choose not to exercise? According to the investigators, a variety of reasons existed, including "family physician disapproval, shift work, lack of interest, simple awareness that such a program existed." Some reflection will suggest that several of these reasons may create noncomparable controls. If, for example, family physicians discourage participation because they fear that the

Table 1.3 Complication Rates for Standard Delivery Versus Alternative
Birthing Center (ABC)

	Standard Delivery (percent of cases)	ABC (percent of cases)
Labor:		
failure to progress	18.3	5.2
C section	9.2	2.3
fetal distress	5.3	0.3
meconium staining	11.9	2.3
Infant:		
child abuse	2.4	0
congenital anomalies	3.0	0.6
jaundice	12.6	2.4

SOURCE: Adapted from Goodlin (1980).

cardiac condition is a contraindication to exercise, or if patients find
exercise objectionable because they are overweight or become
short of breath due to cigarette smoking, differences in experimental group and control group risks could exist. Comparison subjects
may have risk factors that create a greater likelihood of cardiac
death or reinfarction.

A final example may be seen in a study from California that
reported a longitudinal evaluation of the safety of an innovative
approach to childbirth (Goodlin, 1980). The treatment under scrutiny was an alternate birthing center (ABC), a low-technology
environment that features a queen-sized bed, homelike furnish-
ings, and no intravenous drips or fetal monitors. The investigator
wished to learn whether the new center was as safe for mothers
and their newborns as traditional delivery rooms. Some 500 expectant mothers were offered the choice between giving birth in the
standard delivery suite of the hospital or in the new ABC. When
complication rates for mothers and infants in the two groups were
compared, the surprising results shown in Table 1.3 appeared.

The ABC was not *as* safe as the standard delivery room—it was
superior, with much lower rates of such important complications
as failure to progress, C section, and fetal distress; even such
outcomes as congenital anomalies and child abuse were reduced
in the intervention group. That is wonderful news, but there has to
be more here than meets the eye. Why should the delivery site

influence rates of child abuse or congenital anomalies? In all probability, the ABC itself had little to do with the better outcomes. The key is in the self-selection of the subjects who chose this form of delivery. A "healthy volunteer" effect occurs when subjects offer themselves as participants in health experiments, and the women who were willing to try the innovative, low-technology birthing center were likely in a better educated, higher socioeconomic class and were already at lower risk for adverse outcomes than the comparison patients, regardless of the method of delivery.

Conclusion

Issues of control dominate traditional methods of evaluating interventions. The clinical literature is rich in case reports and case-series studies—documents that frequently provide useful clues in the search for more effective treatments but do not solve the case. We can learn whether a new approach to cholecystectomy is technically feasible or if an untried medication shows promise as an antihypertensive. Insights about potential surgical complications or side effects of the drug may be found. But definitive information about treatment efficacy is not a reasonable expectation without explicit comparison subjects. Exhortations in defense of practitioners' clinical trials that it is "both silly and anti-intellectual to ignore or decry all use of historical controls" (Lasagna, 1982) are well intentioned. But history can be capricious. Patient populations change with time; some diseases that beset us are cyclical in nature; some improve spontaneously; regression effects can mimic improvement. If history provides us with one lesson of lasting value, it is that concurrent controls are a necessary part of our evaluations. And, while the participation of well-intentioned volunteers is clearly a boon to clinical research, their healthy constitutions may confound our attempts to achieve non-biased comparisons.

Still, we must continue to test the efficacy of our interventions. If some of our traditional approaches to evaluation have proven to be less than perfect, we are capable of learning from the past. The persistence that clinicians have demonstrated over many years in struggling to improve medical treatments is a useful trait and should ultimately serve us if we can apply that same energy to the rigorous control of our assessments.

References

Balcon, R., Leaver, D., Ross, D., Ross, K., & Sowton, E. (1970). Clinical evaluation of internal mammary artery implantation. *Lancet, 1*, 440-443.

Beecher, H. K. (1955). The powerful placebo. *Journal of the American Medical Association, 59*, 1602-1604.

Benson, H., & McCallie, D. P., Jr. (1979). Angina pectoris and the placebo effect. *New England Journal of Medicine, 300*, 1424-1429.

British Medical Research Council. (1948). Streptomycin treatment of pulmonary tuberculosis. *British Medical Journal, 2*, 4582-4585.

Cohen, I. B. (Ed.). (1941). *Benjamin Franklin's experiments*. Boston: Harvard University Press.

Cousins, N. (1976). Anatomy of an illness (as perceived by the patient). *New England Journal of Medicine, 307*, 1339-1340.

Diehl, H. S., Baker, A. B., & Cowan, D. W. (1938). Cold vaccines: An evaluation based on a controlled study. *Journal of the American Medical Association, 111*(11), 68-73.

Edelstein, L. (1946). William Osler's philosophy. *Bulletin of the History of Medicine, 20*, 292-293.

Franklin, B. (1941). Letter to John Pringle. In I. B. Cohen (Ed.), *Benjamin Franklin's experiments*. Boston: Harvard University Press. (Original letter 1757)

Gehan, E. A., & Freireich, E. J. (1974). Non-randomized controls in cancer clinical trials. *New England Journal of Medicine, 290*, 198-203.

Gehlbach, S. H. (1988). *Interpreting the medical literature* (pp. 107-109). New York: Macmillan.

Goodlin, R. C. (1980). Low-risk obstetric care for low-risk mothers. *Lancet, 1*, 1017-1019.

Langston, M. F., Jr., Kerth, W. J., Selzer, A., & Cohn, K. E. (1972). Evaluation of internal mammary artery implantation. *American Journal of Cardiology, 29*, 788-792.

Lasagna, I. (1982). Historical controls: The practitioner's clinical trials. *New England Journal of Medicine, 307*, 1339-1340.

Leroy, G. V. (1941). The effectiveness of the xanthine drugs in the treatment of angina pectoris. *Journal of the American Medical Association, 116*, 921-925.

Lister, J. (1870). On the effects of the antiseptic system of treatment upon the salubrity of a surgical hospital. *Lancet, 1*, 4-6, 40-42.

Rechnitzer, P. A., Packard, H. A., Pavio, A. U., Yuhasz, M. S., & Cunningham, D. (1972). Long term follow-up study of survival and recurrence rates following myocardial infarction in exercising and control subjects. *Circulation, 45*, 853-856.

Vineberg, A., & Miller, G. (1951). Internal mammary corollary anastomosis in the surgical treatment of coronary artery insufficiency. *Canadian Medical Association Journal, 64*, 204-210.

2 Intervention Studies in Primary Medical Care: Trials and Tribulations

JOHN BAIN

When considering the research methods required in testing ideas for effective intervention in primary care, the backdrop of family practice has to be understood. The laboratory of family practice is the consulting room, where the family physician is faced with patients presenting with a mixture of undifferentiated problems and established diseases. Precision in diagnosis is often lacking, and the physical, psychological, and social factors that influence patients are key features of daily practice. Beyond the consulting room, the delivery of care to patients includes a variety of settings, with the home being the focal point. When continuing care is necessary, a range of health care professionals may be involved in addition to family members. Finally, management of clinical problems has to encompass both an appreciation of patients' understanding of their condition and an appreciation of the determinants of physician behavior in clinical decision making.

When deciding how best to provide care for a specified group of patients, intervention studies have to combine the seeking of infor-

AUTHOR'S NOTE: The research described would not have been possible without the efforts and support of colleagues at Aldermoor Health Centre, Southampton. Dr. Peter Burke and Dr. Kevin Jones have made major contributions to the work on middle ear disorders and asthma, and the advice from Dr. Anne-Louise Kinmonth and Dr. Elizabeth Murphy was particularly valuable during the various stages of the projects. Thanks are also due to all the research assistants who were involved in the projects described.

mation about patients' concerns with attempts to identify sub-groups of those at special risk.

Reports of original work tend to focus on precision of the methods used, tabulated results, and clinical interpretation of the study described. It is seldom that they highlight where the original ideas *came* from, the development of the methods relevant to the setting of the studies, or the ongoing process of the projects. This chapter describes some research that dealt with two common problems in family practice, middle ear disorders and asthma, to illustrate how important questions in primary care can be tackled.

Background of the Research Projects

Middle ear disorders in children and asthma affecting all age groups are two of the most common conditions seen by family physicians. The prevalence of the former has been estimated at between 10% and 15% in children under 10 years of age, with the condition particularly common in the preschool and early school years. In the United Kingdom, asthma affects about 11% of children in this age group and about 8% of individuals of all ages.

Middle Ear Disorders

In day-to-day discussion in our practice at Aldermoor Health Centre, and in talking to a wide range of local family physicians, the problems of management of earache in children were frequently brought to the fore. Questions included these: Are decongestant-antihistamine mixtures effective? Do the parents ensure that a recommended course of treatment is completed? Are antibiotics always necessary?

In designing studies to try and answer these questions, the first step was to learn more about current diagnostic and prescribing behaviors. An examination of symptoms recorded by 25 family physicians in 1,137 children with new episodes of respiratory and ear disorders revealed a wide range of presenting symptomatology. "Presumed middle ear infection" stood out as the condition where the percentage of children with individual symptoms was higher for a larger range of symptoms than any of the other

Table 2.1 Range of Presenting Symptoms in Children Given a
Diagnosis of Acute Otitis Media (N = 239 cases of AOM)

Symptom	Percent
Fever	34
Loss of appetite	33
Crying	40
Unwell	50
Sore throat	15
Nasal discharge	61
Cough	55
Night cough	42
Earache	77
Earache at night	48

respiratory conditions (see Table 2.1). In addition, a variety of
statements were used to describe the findings on ear examination
(see Table 2.2).

The main lesson from this preliminary study was that family
physicians were dealing here with symptom-sign complexes;
hence any studies that were to be relevant to management would
have to be based on the reality of daily practice.

Between 1980 and 1988, a succession of studies was set up to
answer three specific questions regarding the primary care treatment of acute otitis media:

1. Can its clinical course be modified by systemic decongestant or
   antihistamine treatment?
2. Is a short course of antibiotic treatment as effective as the traditional
   7- to 10-day course?
3. Are antibiotics essential at all?

The detailed design and results of these studies have been reported elsewhere (Bain, 1983; Bain, Murphy, & Ross, 1985; Burke,
Bain, Robinson, & Dunleavy, 1991; Jones & Bain, 1986). A cursory
description is presented below, with a focus on how the participating physicians were involved in the studies and what they learned
from them.

Table 2.2 Ear Drum Examination: List of Variables Recorded by Family
Physicians

R. Ear Drum	Visualized	L. Ear Drum
	Normal	
	Uniform redness	
	Pink blush/prominent	
	blood vessels	
	Injection handle malleus	
	Red rim	
	Bulging drum	
	Drum indrawn	
	Drum perforated	
	Discharge	
	Loss light reflex	
	(Other)	

OWNERSHIP OF THE IDEAS

The original ideas emanated from individuals with a special
interest in the subject; however, all the physicians who participated
in the studies were included at early stages of the discussions about
research method and design. A total of 102 family practitioners
(Study I: 24; Study II: 30; Study III: 48) were recruited and, throughout the projects, attended a series of workshops where methods
were discussed and progress reported. The number of children
entered in the study by each physician varied, but all physicians
retained an ongoing interest and commitment. It was apparent that
the studies related to issues that presented them with dilemmas in
management, and meeting to discuss the stages of the project not
only gave them continuing insight into the problems of conducting
research but, more important, provided a sense of ownership of the
project.

DESIGN OF THE STUDIES AND THEIR PROGRESS

1. Given that the preliminary work had demonstrated that family physicians were dealing with symptom-sign complexes, an
encounter form was designed that would reflect their experiences

of presenting problems rather than forcing physicians to agree on a rigid definition of otitis media.

In effect, the studies were about how to deal with a child presenting with "painful red ears." At a series of workshops, descriptive terms for eardrum signs were agreed to, with the aid of a standard set of slides. Here again, the participating physicians were "in on the take-offs and landings" of the design of the studies.

2. Small pilot studies were conducted with parents who agreed to help with the design of the studies and give advice about the content of diary cards that would be used by them to assess their children's progress.

3. It was clear that office reception staff would be key players in the studies. Accordingly, a study coordinator ensured that they were briefed about the nature of the study and their specific responsibilities in arranging follow-up and issuing trial drugs.

4. Statistical advice was sought early, and this provided the required information about sample size. A statistician was also involved in the design of the recording cards, to ensure adequate analysis of results.

5. Family physicians are busy people; thus the recordings that they had to make at entry to the study and at a follow-up consultation (one week later) were kept to a minimum. Once a child had been entered in the study, parental consent obtained, and the record form completed, the parents were instructed to obtain from reception staff both the diary cards for following their child's progress and the appropriate drugs.

6. More detailed follow-up of the children's progress to ensure that their parents both understood the project and were complying with instructions was conducted by two trained research assistants (for each study) who paid regular visits to the children's homes. These assistants assessed children at 1 month and 3 months after entry, when tympanometry was executed.

7. For all three studies, it was agreed that the age range for inclusion would be restricted to 3 to 10 years, because younger children present special difficulties in communication and assessment and require varying doses of drugs.

RESULTS AND OUTCOME

1. By spending considerable time with all the participants, it was possible to reduce problem areas to a minimum. Fewer than 10%

of children in all three studies failed to complete the trials (the reasons are provided in the published reports).

2. Few doctors discontinued involvement. Those who continued throughout the trials did so largely because they were very interested in the outcome.

3. Parents in all socioeconomic groups maintained interest in the studies, presumably because they were well informed about why the studies were being carried out and because their children received considerable attention throughout the studies.

4. In Study I, a follow-up over a 2-month period showed that there was no significant difference in terms of resolution of symptoms associated with presumed acute otitis media (eardrum signs, recurrence, or hospital referral) between pseudoephedrine, triprolidine, and placebo.

In Study II, resolution of symptoms at days 1, 5, and 10 showed no significant differences between a 2-day, high-dose course of antibiotic compared with the conventional dosage for 7 days.

5. In Study III, treatment failure during the first week was eight times more frequent in the placebo group (14.4% versus 1.7%), and children in this group showed a higher analgesic consumption, a greater duration of crying, and longer absence from school. Longer-term outcomes in terms of recurrence, referral to hospital, and abnormal tympanograms were not significantly different in the antibiotic and placebo groups.

IMPACT

1. The most notable impact of these studies on the treatment of presumed otitis media was the reduction in use of decongestant-antihistamine drugs by U.K. family physicians. This was partly due to a government decision to withdraw the majority of these drugs from the "prescription list" following the results of this study being taken into consideration by an expert panel.

2. It is more difficult to judge the extent to which family physicians in general now use a short course of antibiotics instead of the traditional 7- to 10-day course. There can be little doubt, however, that those doctors who participated in the study were strongly influenced by the results.

3. All those participating in the studies (parents, receptionists, researchers, and doctors) became more aware of the need to conduct original work both in the setting of the family physician's

office and in patient homes. The main lesson to be learned was that a successful outcome in terms of completing the projects was dependent on a team effort, where *all* those involved were informed from the beginning of the project about its aims, with regular feedback sessions to maintain interest and enthusiasm.

4. Study III (the antibiotic-placebo trial) is likely to reassure the majority of family physicians that the use of antibiotics in treating presumed acute otitis media is generally justified. For those who choose a "wait-and-see policy," however, there is evidence that the long-term outcome for children not treated is not adversely affected.

OVERALL OUTCOME

This succession of trials showed how controlled randomized clinical trials can be conducted in general practice. The methods used to record information did not go beyond the boundaries of the family physicians' regular assessment of children presenting with "painful red ears."

The research team consisted of a small core of five committed researchers (two physicians and three research assistants) for each study, but the extended team included all the participating physicians and their support staffs. By spreading the load around 20-40 doctors, the extra work involved in recruiting patients was not excessive.

There are limitations to these studies as the patients studied may not be representative of all children in that age group. They do, however, represent that group of ear problems where moderate symptoms and signs present difficulties for doctors when faced with dilemmas over management decisions.

The costs of these studies, in terms of both time allocation and money required to employ support staff, were not substantial in comparison with costs incurred in large, multicentered, laboratory-based research. The overall costs (research staff, equipment, data analysis) were in the region of £75,000.

The next steps in this field of original work will be to refine methods of measuring the beliefs and values of parents, family physicians, and hospital specialists when faced with children with middle ear disorders.

Table 2.3 Parents' Knowledge of Asthma and Purpose of Treatments
($N = 50$)

Area of Knowledge	Percent
Adequate understanding of asthma	20
Adequate understanding of treatment	58
Know about possibility of lung damage	68
Know that death could occur	70
Had feared death in their children	95
Know danger signs of severe asthma	10

Asthma

It is now well recognized that, despite recent advances in the understanding of the pathogenesis of asthma and despite the new treatments and delivery systems available, morbidity and mortality rates are not falling (Burney, 1986; Evans et al., 1987; Mayo, Semenciw, & Morrison, 1987). There have been several recent calls for the improvement of asthma management in primary care in the United Kingdom. In talking to family physicians and their support staffs, however, it was clear that several issues had to be considered before designing intervention studies to raise standards of care.

One thing that became apparent was that it was necessary to explore patients' understanding of this condition. Parents' knowledge about their children's asthma was chosen as the starting point. A small study was conducted in one health center where 50 children aged 5-10 years with established asthma (on continuous treatment) were identified. A simple questionnaire was designed to determine their parents' knowledge of the disorder and the purpose of treatments. The results, shown in Table 2.3, highlight the problems of inadequate understanding. Based on these findings, Study I was designed to answer the question: Could understanding and self-management be improved, with benefits occurring in terms of lung function and daily living?

An asthma clinic offering further education and instruction in inhaler technique was subsequently set up for all patients in one practice, and a parallel study on both children and adults was designed to test the hypothesis that patients' understanding and improvements in lung function and daily activities can be enhanced by structured care within a group practice.

Asthma is an extremely common condition (around 8% of the population), so the task of following up all asthmatics in one practice is a considerable one. After these preliminary studies in one practice, the questions that now arose were these:

1. Could the extent of asthma be measured in a variety of practices?
2. Could we develop a disability index that would identify those patients most at risk and requiring more detailed intervention?

These questions led to Study II, in which three family practices in the south of England, with a total of 20,100 patients and 16 physicians, were selected for study. Asthmatic patients were identified from computerized repeat-prescribing registers, and 100 patients in each practice aged between 5 and 65 years were randomly selected from those so identified.

The patients identified were then interviewed and completed an extended questionnaire derived from previously tested instruments (Hilton, Sibbald, Anderson, & Freeling, 1982). Also at this time, inhaler technique was scored and lung function measured using a turbine spirometer (Jones & Middleton, 1989).

In both studies, the issues of *ownership, study design,* and *results and outcome* were again assessed throughout.

OWNERSHIP OF THE IDEAS

Concern about asthma care was widespread during the time in which these studies were being conducted. The driving forces for conducting Study I came from just two people (a doctor and a nurse practitioner), but the whole practice became involved in the process of obtaining information, following up the patients, and sharing results. Consequently, there was an overall commitment to making attempts to improve care of asthmatic patients. With the subsequent departure from the practice of the two initiators, there was a fear that the impetus would be lost; however, to date, it appears that this practice has retained its interest in asthma care, with a treatment room nurse continuing to offer services.

In Study II, the extended study in three practices, it was agreed at an early stage that, in addition to collecting information about asthma patients, the research team would help the practices maintain a register of the patients and give advice and support in setting up structured systems of follow-up care. This has cemented the team's relationship with these practices and has not made staff there feel as if they were merely being used as settings for data collection.

An extremely important aspect of "ownership" was identified in Study I, where the development of self-management plans enabled patients to take responsibility for their own conditions. A combination of regular review by the family physician and a structured self-management plan has allowed shared care to occur (Charlton, Charlton, Broomfield, & Mullee, 1990).

DESIGN OF THE STUDIES AND THEIR PROGRESS

1. The participants in the study were brought in at an early stage, where aims and objectives were clearly set out.

2. Staff at all levels of the primary care team were invited to a series of meetings throughout the projects, and their views were actively sought about the extent to which they could be involved in collecting information.

3. Regular contacts occurred between the researchers and the reception staff, nurses, and family physicians. This ensured that information gathered from patients' records was understood and that visits to patients only occurred after they had received and acknowledged a letter from their own family physician.

4. This close contact between researchers and practice teams allowed for identification of patients who would be unsuitable for inclusion in the projects. In Study II, 18 subjects were found to be unsuitable for interview because of concurrent illness and other life events, and these individuals were not approached.

5. The methods for selecting and analyzing results were discussed regularly with a statistician, who became an integral part of the research team.

6. The studies did not impose any burdens on the family physicians or their support staffs to collect any additional information when consulted by asthmatic patients. The conduct of the single clinic in Study I, and the interviews and assessments in Study II, were all carried out by members of the research team.

7. Regular feedback sessions occurred in which problem areas were ironed out and modifications to the study design discussed. In Study II, the physicians were kept fully up to date about when interviews with patients would be taking place.

RESULTS AND OUTCOME

1. The overall results of Study I, which included 115 patients in one practice, demonstrated that teaching patients about the importance of their symptoms and the appropriate action to be taken when their asthma condition deteriorates were the keys to effective management of their condition (Charlton et al., 1990).

2. In Study II, 296 of 300 patients in these practices completed the project—testimony to their cooperation and to the support of their family physicians.

3. The collection of detailed information about daily activities and lung function required a long-standing commitment from both the research staff and the practices over a 4-year period.

4. The results pertaining to asthma morbidity and lung function in Study II are shown in Tables 2.4 and 2.5 and again highlight the extent to which this condition impinges on daily living. An important outcome was the development of a morbidity index (Table 2.6). (For details of how this index was calculated, see Jones, Bain, Middleton, & Mullee, 1992.) This study did not include specific interventions to modify asthma care. Its main aim was to "fingerprint" how intervention was applied and to develop an instrument that could be used for future intervention studies.

IMPACT

1. In the self-management study, there was ample evidence that the main impact was on patients' understanding of their condition. The concept of "shared" rather than "dependent" care has relevance to a variety of chronic conditions in primary care.

2. In both studies, the family physicians and their support staffs became much more aware of the need to develop methods to identify asthmatic patients, to make arrangements for regular review, and to draw up practice policies for care.

Table 2.4 Morbidity in Patients with Asthma ($N = 296$)

Characteristics	Number	Percent
Wheezy or asthmatic condition at least once per week?	145	49
Asthma/wheezing interrupts daily life at least monthly?	33	11
Avoid mild exercise between attacks?	13	4
Avoid energetic sports between attacks?	56	19
Avoid parties and social gatherings between attacks?	18	6
Everyday activities affected quite a lot or a great deal in past 12 months?	28	10
Asthma worse in past year?	46	16
*Stayed off work or school because of asthma:		
ever?	151	60
in past year?	77	31
Attacks of wheezing during night?	150	51
When wakened, sleep again with difficulty or not at all?	52	17
Current smokers?	41	14
Ex-regular smokers?	35	31
Passive smokers?	96	32
Pets?		
Number of homes with pets:		
Total	191	65
Dogs	107	36
Cats	68	23
Birds	31	12

*$N = 250$ (46 do not go to work or school).

3. Involvement of receptionists and nurses as well as physicians in the research process has heightened their desire for more knowledge, and there is ample evidence that a team approach to the care of chronic conditions is beginning to emerge.

Table 2.5 Lung Function in Patients with Asthma ($N = 296$)

Lung Function	n	Mean (SD)
FEV 1 as percentage of predicted:	259	66.9 (18.4)
FVC as percentage of predicted:	259	81.1 (18.9)
PEFR as percentage of predicted:	284	79.9 (18.9)
Amplitude percentage mean:	284	24.2 (17.4)

Table 2.6 Morbidity Index

Question

Are you in a wheezy or asthmatic condition at least once per week?
Have you had time off work or school in the last year because of your asthma?
Do you suffer from attacks of wheezing during the night?

NOTE: "No" to all 3 questions = low morbidity; 1 "Yes" = medium morbidity; and "Yes" to 2
or 3 = high morbidity.

4. For the clinicians, there is now an instrument (the morbidity
index) that can help them decide on priorities in patient care. In the
midst of constant demands to improve the quality of care in family
practice, it is impossible to extend its horizons beyond certain
limits and, in the case of asthma, there are groups of patients who
probably require closer attention than others. Intervention studies
are still required to scrutinize the effectiveness of the morbidity
index, but, from the results obtained, it appears to be sufficiently
robust to be used as an aid in daily practice.

OVERALL OUTCOME

It is too early to judge the overall outcome of these initial studies
of asthma, but there is no doubt that there is now a heightened
awareness among family physicians and other members of the
primary care team about the importance of this condition. Patients
are now in a better position to understand how they can "take
charge" of their condition, and there are possibilities for the use of
the morbidity index in future intervention studies.

Members of the research team are now much in demand to
conduct workshops and give lectures to primary care professionals
throughout the United Kingdom. The core research staff included
three family physicians and three research assistants; but, as with
the studies on middle ear disorders, the extended team of researchers included a wide variety of primary care staff in the practices
included in the studies.

The research costs over a 5-year period were in the region of
£120,000. For the extent of the work involved, this was not excessive, given that the core staff were involved in daily practice as well.
The next step in this work will be to test the morbidity index on a

wider scale as well as to facilitate the process whereby practices can conduct their own intervention studies in the care of asthmatic patients.

Conclusions

Many of the "trials and tribulations" encountered in these studies are difficult to put down on paper. The intervention studies relating to management of presumed middle ear infection relied on the tried-and-tested methods of the randomized controlled trial. There are limitations to all trials because human beings are not like plants in a pot, and controlling all extraneous variables simply is not possible. The human factor was nowhere more apparent than in the situations faced by research assistants when they were used as sounding boards for family problems. On some occasions, interviewers were not sure whether to pass on information to the patients' family physicians, and this raised problems about confidentiality. These experiences emphasized that there is often a conflict between collection of data and putting the patient's needs first (Murphy, 1985).

The research methods reported relied not only on statistical advice regarding required numbers and methods of randomization but on the collaboration of physicians who saw the questions posed as worthy of testing. Their ongoing interest and commitment were maintained by regular communication and attention to detail. Informal discussions with the many practitioners who took part indicated that they found it helpful to have objective measurements of their clinical performance. They also indicated that the findings of these clinical trials of treatment regimens relating to the *symptoms* and *signs* of middle ear disorders have resulted in a more widespread discussion about conventional methods of prescribing (Aylett, 1990; Browning, 1990; Hurwitz, Acheson, Steel, & Carney, 1984).

The work on the nature of asthmatic patients was of a more exploratory nature but was necessary before embarking on more widespread interventions. Like *otitis media*, the term *asthma* includes a broad spectrum of problems relating not only to the respiratory tract but to other features of patient behavior. While accepting that precision in diagnosis remains the cornerstone of much of clinical practice, a collection of symptoms and physical signs does not always constitute a recognized disease but may be a cue for action (Marinker, 1982, in Cormack, Marinker, & Morrell, 1982). This is true in the case of asthma, where there is still debate about the natural history of the condition. Accordingly, entry to the studies was simply based on the prescribing of "antiasthma" drugs, with no attempt to force family physicians into narrow definitions for their patients' presenting problems.

It was clear from the start of the research on asthma that the nature and severity of the condition varied considerably, both between age groups and between patients in similar age groups. A point was reached where it was necessary to attempt to categorize patients in terms of their level of morbidity before pursuing active intervention projects. There were many "trials and tribulations" and "false starts" before agreement was reached about the actual methods to be adopted. Again, regular discussion with family physicians and their support staffs ensured that everyone involved was conversant with the aims of the study. In addition to gaining new knowledge about potential approaches to management, the members of the practices taking part became more aware of their own needs in terms of organizing care for asthmatic patients. This latter outcome probably has had, to date, as important an impact as the creation of a morbidity index; and this example of "action research" can serve as a model for those wishing to integrate research workers with those in full-time practice.

It is worth noting that none of the participating physicians received payment for taking part in these projects, and their commitment was based on the efforts made by the research team to include their views throughout the progress of all the projects.

There are many lessons to be learned from the projects reported here. The dominant research values in medicine still largely focus on rare conditions and pathologies, which are not perceived as d'rectly applicable to the family physician. Research into common clinical problems, with outcomes based on original work in family practice, is needed if the results are to be relevant to family physicians.

Central to any work that has to be conducted in a family practice setting are the themes of *ownership of the ideas, design of studies*, and *their progress and impact on clinical practice*. By raising awareness about these themes, collaboration between researchers and full-time clinicians can be enhanced, and the "trials and tribulations" of conducting original work can be shared by all those participating in the work.

References

Aylett, M. (1990). Acute otitis media. *British Medical Journal, 300,* 1341-1342.

Bain, J. (1983). Can the clinical course of acute otitis media be modified by systemic decongestant or anti-histamine treatment? *British Medical Journal, 287,* 654-656.

Bain, J., Murphy, E., & Ross, F. (1985). Acute otitis media: Clinical course among children who received a short course of high dose antibiotic. *British Medical Journal, 291,* 1243-1246.

Browning, G. G. (1990). Controversies in therapeutics: Childhood otalgia: Acute otitis media. Antibiotics not necessary in most cases. *British Medical Journal, 300,* 1005-1006.

Burke, P., Bain, J., Robinson, D., & Dunleavy, J. (1991). Acute red ear in children: Controlled trial of non-antibiotic treatment in general practice. *British Medical Journal, 303,* 558-561.

Burney, P. G. J. (1986). Asthma mortality in England and Wales: Evidence for a further increase. *Lancet, 2,* 323-326.

Charlton, I., Charlton, G., Broomfield, J., & Mullee, M. A. (1990). Evaluation of peak flow and symptoms only self management plans for control of asthma in general practice. *British Medical Journal, 301,* 1355-1359.

Cormack, J., Marinker, M., & Morrell, D. (Eds.). (1982). *Practice: A handbook of primary medical care.* London: Kluwer Medical.

Evans, R., Mullally, D. I., Wilson, R. W., Gergen, P. J., Rosenberg, H. M., Grauman, J. S., Chevarley, F. M., & Feinleib, M. (1987). National trends in the morbidity and mortality of asthma in the U.S. *Chest, 91,* 65-74.

Hilton, S., Sibbald, B., Anderson, H. R., & Freeling, P. (1982). Evaluating health education in asthma: Developing the methodology. *Journal of the Royal Society of Medicine, 75,* 625-630.

Hurwitz, B., Acheson, H. W. K., Steel, A. M., & Carney, T. A. (1984). Response to paper on "Can the clinical course of acute otitis media be modified by systemic decongestant or anti-histamine treatment." *British Medical Journal, 288,* 977-979.

Jones, K., & Middleton, M. (1989, June). Benefits of an inhaler-technique scoring system. *Update, 38*(12), 1399-1403.

Jones, K., Bain, J., Middleton, M., & Mullee, M. A. (1992). Correlates of asthma morbidity in primary care. *British Medical Journal, 304,* 361-364.

Jones, R., & Bain, J. (1986). Three day and seven day treatment in acute otitis media: A double-blind antibiotic trial. *Journal of the Royal College of General Practitioners, 36,* 356-358.

Mayo, Y., Semenciw, R., & Morrison, H. (1987). Increased rates of illness and death from asthma in Canada. *Canadian Medical Association Journal, 137,* 620-624.

Murphy, E. A. (1985). Practical considerations in conducting research in primary medical care. *British Medical Journal, 291,* 577-578.

PART II

Two Major Approaches
to Assessing Interventions
in Primary Care

This part of the volume considers two major methods of inquiry in the primary care setting—quantitative and qualitative methodologies, the former of which is commonly associated with clinical research, and the latter with either "soft" data or with nonmedical disciplines such as anthropology. Four chapters are devoted to each method: one to theory, two to examples, and the last to discussing application of methods to primary care.

For the quantitative section, Dr. Fletcher, an editor and international writer on epidemiological methodology, discusses the use of randomized trials. He presents several key issues that he believes need to be addressed: targeted studies, strong studies of real-life practice, blinding, measurements, negative trials, and units of analysis.

Dr. Labrecque, an academic family physician, and Professor Mohide, an academic nurse-researcher, present investigations of their own that provide examples of randomized trials in primary care settings. In both cases, their work produced negative findings, yet the results prove as useful as if they had been positive. The description of the "trials and tribulations" encountered in their respective studies may be the most valuable part of their contributions.

To close the quantitative section, Dr. Donner, a professor of epidemiology and biostatistics, reflects on the issues that were introduced by Dr. Fletcher and illustrated in Dr. Labrecque's and Professor Mohide's examples. In particular, he raises several issues that are important with respect to running trials in primary care settings: the nature of the intervention, the control group, and the trial setting; the interpretation of nonsignificant results; and the choice of unit of analysis.

The second set of four chapters deals with issues of qualitative designs. It opens with a discussion by Dr. Jenkins, an academic in both anthropology and psychiatry, which contrasts the qualitative versus the quantitative ways of knowing, in particular within the "culture" of primary care. To illustrate, she describes her own work on the relationship between expressed emotion and clinical outcome and the importance that communication has for the doctor-patient interaction.

Dr. Willms, a researcher in both clinical epidemiology and anthropology, recounts how a study of smoking cessation caused him to reconsider how to conduct such interventions and then describes his qualitative methods of analysis, which hinge on examining patients' expressed words. Dr. Seifert, a community family physician, tells us how he integrates qualitative clinical research with patient care by viewing patients as coresearchers and the practice as a laboratory setting, through setting up focus groups of his own patients.

Finally, Dr. Good, an internationally recognized qualitative researcher, discusses the three previous chapters in light of what she refers to as "a meaning-centered approach" to research in primary care. Her discussion walks us through the leading edge of qualitative methodologies in primary care today: research issues such as understanding of illness realities and the narrative aspect of physician-patient interactions.

Together, these eight chapters exemplify work that is building on our knowledge of the two primary methodological paths for primary care research—work that is significant and relevant to the field because it comes from clinical experience.

3 Randomized Trials
for Assessing Interventions
in Primary Care

ROBERT H. FLETCHER

As primary care physicians, all of the good that we may do is ultimately effected through some sort of intervention. Some of these interventions are similar to those offered by other branches of medicine; for example, prescribing medications or performing minor surgery. Others are more characteristic of our specialties (though not unique to them): giving advice and reassurance, teaching, screening, immunizing, and early detection.

It is by no means the case that every intervention in day-to-day use is effective. Effectiveness is relatively easy to establish for treatment of disorders that have a single, dominant cause and short-term outcomes, such as antibiotics for gonococcal urethritis or bronchodilators for acute asthma. But many conditions that primary care physicians attempt to prevent or alleviate (for example, cardiovascular disease or cancer, anxiety or depression) have many interacting causes and remote, probabilistic effects. For these, it is difficult to tell through personal experience whether an intervention, however well intentioned or conventional, truly does more good than harm.

How can we know whether our efforts work? We look to many forms of support for our actions, some of them intellectual and some emotional; certainly not all are of equal value (Fletcher, 1990). We may believe our efforts work because we want them to work, because our seniors advocate them, or because they ought to work according to our understanding of the mechanisms of disease. All these are forms of justification, but they can take us off track. (How many of them, after all, are also the rationales of witch doctors and faith healers?) As one author put it, "We should do things not because they ought to work, but because they do work" (Anonymous, 1980).

The best evidence for the effectiveness of an intervention comes from properly conducted randomized controlled trials (RCTs), whereby patients with the condition of interest are randomly allocated to receive either the treatment under investigation or an alternative one (the usual treatment or, if none is known to be effective, a placebo). The randomization assures us that on average the two groups would have a similar prognosis if treated the same way, and so is a way of isolating the effects of the intervention from the many other factors that could affect outcome. The two groups are observed over time, then the rates of outcome events are measured and compared. If the rates in the groups are different, and if this difference is unlikely to have occurred by chance and is large enough to be clinically important, then we have an answer: The treatment works. If the rates are so similar that any observed differences could easily be by chance, and the largest plausible difference consistent with the data is still not clinically important, then we also have an answer: The treatment does not work (Braitman, 1991).

There are excellent monographs on how to conduct randomized controlled trials (Friedman, Furberg, & DeMets, 1985; Pocock, 1983) and also textbooks of clinical epidemiology that describe how to judge and interpret clinical trials published in the medical literature (Fletcher, Fletcher, & Wagner, 1988; Sackett, Haynes, Guyett, & Tugwell, 1991). This chapter discusses how general principles of clinical trial design, conduct, and analysis can be adapted to the special needs of primary care.

Randomized Controlled Trials Versus Alternatives

RCTs are the most scientifically credible way to characterize the effects of an intervention and are relatively easy to design; however, they are difficult to carry out. One must assemble a large number of patients, persuade them to receive treatment of unknown value, follow them over time, and have them undergo special examinations to assess the outcomes. All of this takes resources—money, time, effort—that are in limited supply for most primary care physicians. As a result, there are many more clinically important questions than there are resources to answer them.

There do exist alternatives to RCTs that are more practical to carry out, but these are also, unfortunately, less scientifically valid. In *cohort studies*, patients with the condition of interest are assembled at some uniform point in the course of their disease. Some happen to get the experimental treatment as part of ordinary patient care, and others do not. Treatment decisions are made as clinical decisions, and not by random assignment. All are followed forward in time, and the rates of outcomes in the two groups are compared. At their best, cohort studies are similar to well-done RCTs in all important respects except for randomization (Feinstein, 1983). In *case control studies*, rates of exposure to the intervention are compared in people with or without the outcome. The rates are used to estimate the relative risk of experiencing the outcome in the two groups—that is, to estimate the effectiveness of treatment. Case control studies are relatively inexpensive and fast but also vulnerable to many biases that must be dealt with carefully.

The challenges faced by all research designs other than RCTs are that the experimental intervention is never the only determinant of outcome and the other determinants are not necessarily distributed equally in treatment groups. This situation leads to confounding, where another cause for the outcome is mistaken for the one being studied. In the absence of randomization, it is necessary to find some other way of comparing like with like. The options include restricting the sample of patients studied to those with a narrow range of characteristics, matching patients in the treated group with patients of similar characteristics in the control group, analyzing the data within groups ("strata") of similar characteristics, mathematical modeling, or some combination of these (Fletcher et al., 1988).

RCTs in Primary Care

More RCT studies are badly needed in primary care, because too many interventions in day-to-day practice are being undertaken without sound knowledge of their effectiveness. Most published clinical trials are done by subspecialist physicians in referral centers and, as a result, their findings are not generalizable to primary care practice. The diseases they address are usually uncommon, unlike primary care conditions; the patients who take part in them have traversed a long referral chain, making them quite unlike those seen by first-contact physicians; the interventions performed may not be available in office practice; and the outcomes are usually strictly biological, excluding the clinical and human outcomes valued by primary care physicians and their patients.

Clinical trials in the primary care setting are based on the same principles as those in more specialized settings; however, they have a distinct profile of advantages and challenges. The most obvious advantage is that they deal with relatively common conditions, making it easier to gather enough patients and to detect clinically important differences for the main outcomes—and perhaps even for subgroups—without resort to collaborative, multicenter arrangements and great expense. That is, it is relatively easy to achieve a large sample size and high statistical power and precision. (An exception is trials of preventive interventions, where outcomes are expected to be uncommon and long after the intervention.)

There are other advantages. Primary care physicians are used to working in teams, as one usually must do for clinical trials. They may have fewer dropouts from trials, because they know their patients well. Studies in the primary care setting are closer to the realities of day-to-day patient care than are subspecialty studies and so can be generalized to a larger array of other settings. Finally, the field is relatively unworked; anything that is done well is likely to be welcome.

Along with these advantages, there are also special challenges for those who would do RCTs in primary care settings. These are not necessarily problems but issues to be grappled with, choices to be made.

TARGETED STUDIES

Primary care physicians are generalists by choice and by training and hold a holistic view of illness, its causes, and management. This may make it difficult for them to design scientifically credible trials, for the following reasons. First, given their view that disease is caused by many factors in the biological, physical, and social environment, and that these factors are related to each other in complex ways, they may find it artificial to study the effects of one factor while holding the others constant. Yet, if they will not see clinical problems in a more restricted way, they cannot design trials with enough internal validity to be reasonably sure that the results are true.

Similarly, they may believe that all interventions should have many dimensions—for example, advice, diet, medications, and reassurance—and so find it awkward to examine the effects of just one or two alone. They may believe that nonspecific (placebo) effects are an important part of their armamentarium, responsible for much of the healing they can offer. Yet clinical trials often compare new treatments with placebos, subtracting out the placebo effect.

Finally, RCTs ordinarily focus on one or just a few outcomes, whereas primary care physicians concern themselves with many outcomes, ranging from biological to psychological, social, and economic. For example, the outcomes of treating mild hypertension are not confined to blood pressure (and ultimately stroke, congestive heart failure, and renal failure) but may also include fatigue, impotence, cost, and perhaps increased risk for other diseases such as diabetes and hyperlipidemia.

The point is not which worldview—holistic versus reductionistic—is right or wrong. I happen to believe that the more complex view that is characteristic of primary care is closer to clinical reality. Convincing clinical trials, however, cannot be done under an entirely holistic view, and, without RCTs, hypotheses about interventions are not put to a strong test. Primary care physicians must give some ground to the reductionistic point of view to accomplish good science. They must look at one or at most a small number of kinds of patients, interventions, and outcomes at a time. The complexity can then be addressed by doing more trials with other patients, interventions, and outcomes and building up the general picture through multiple restricted studies, each sound in its own right. It is a discouraging compromise, one that many primary care physicians have been unwilling to make. But it is part of the nature of scientific inquiry, and there can be no progress in scientific terms without it.

STRONG STUDIES OF REAL-LIFE PRACTICES

A second challenge is how to make the trade-off between trials of highly selected patients in relatively artificial settings to maximize the *internal validity* of the study ("efficacy trials") and trials of more ordinary patients in ordinary settings to maximize *generalizability* ("effectiveness trials"). Most published trials lean toward the former. They are about unusual patients, chosen to have a definite diagnosis of a specific disease—yet most patients' conditions are not so clear-cut. Most trials will exclude patients who have other diseases—yet in practice many patients do have other diseases. And, of course, patients in RCTs are expected to cooperate and to avoid potential biases, noncompliance with treatment, and loss to follow-up; however, this leaves out large numbers of patients (such as the poor, elderly, or drug dependent) who cannot. Because of these entry and exclusion criteria, it is not uncommon for investigators to screen hundreds of potentially eligible patients to enter just one. Such trials are then poorly generalizable to ordinary practice and especially to primary care practice, which is where most patients receive care.

The problem with conducting trials with fewer of these restrictions is that there is a penalty to pay in the form of decreased internal validity; that is, the results may be less believable. For example, if the patients have less classic disease, and some may not even have the disease at all, they are more heterogeneous; this introduces more "noise" into the system being studied, making it more difficult to detect the "signal"—the specific effects of the intervention. Real-life patients may drop out of the study or cross over to the other treatment, and, if this occurs on a large scale, it makes the results uninterpretable. Real-world clinicians often tailor treatments to individual patients, and their patients expect this, yet this makes the intervention less reproducible.

The trade-off between internal validity and generalizability cannot be avoided, and there is no single right answer as to where it should be made. Some scholars believe that too many RCTs nowadays are unbalanced in favor of internal validity and so are not useful guides for the practice of medicine. The challenge is to find ways to conduct trials that more closely match the real world while still retaining enough scientific strength. For example, one might increase sample size to make up for heterogeneity and to allow

enough statistical power to look for effects within clinically meaningful subgroups. Or, one might make special efforts to follow up
patients who have dropped out in cases where outcomes would be
apparent even without patients' cooperation. As for compliance
with the therapeutic regimen, this is a downstream consequence of
the intervention; by analyzing patients according to the group they
were randomized to, not to the one who received treatment, one
has a study of the policy of *recommending* treatment, whether or not
it is taken (Sackett et al., 1991).

BLINDING

In an ideal trial (from a purely scientific point of view), there is
complete "blinding" of participants, whereby researchers assign
patients to treatments without knowing who got what, and none
of the patients, the physicians treating them, or whoever assesses
the outcomes knows which treatment each person has received.
The purpose of all this is to remove the possibility of bias in the
comparison—systematic differences that could arise because of
knowledge of treatment group.

In clinical trials of drugs, blinding is ordinarily accomplished by
giving control patients an intervention (a placebo) that is indistin-
guishable from the active treatment in color, taste, texture, and
route of administration. Even in these trials, it is more often claimed
than accomplished, because blinding of this ideal sort is rarely
possible. Trials sometimes approach the ideal, but the treatment
group is often disclosed by physiological or adverse effects of the
active treatment (for example, bradycardia with beta-blockers or
nausea with cholestyramine). Whatever the reason, as a practical
matter, patients can often guess correctly, at the end of even well-
conducted trials, which treatment they have received. Moreover,
many interventions, including most that are important to primary
care, cannot be blinded at all. Among these are minor surgery,
diets, advice, and reassurance. Unfortunately, bias arising from
knowledge of treatment group is likely to affect the outcomes that
are most important.

Because complete blinding is usually not possible in primary
care trials, researchers must be especially meticulous in those
aspects of it that are within their control: assignment of treatment and measurement of outcomes. They must also exert careful

quality control on the remaining aspects by means of operational definitions of outcomes and careful records of treatments actually received and of other interventions that might have affected outcomes.

MEASUREMENTS

Many of the outcomes of primary care are difficult to measure. We hope that our patients will, partly as a result of our efforts, suffer less discomfort (e.g., pain, nausea, dyspnea, anxiety, loneliness) and have less limitation of function. These outcomes often cannot be verified directly with the physical senses or with laboratory instruments as can such phenomena as tumor regression, renal function, oxygenation, or markers of inflammatory disease. One must find indirect ways of measuring them—which is why they are called "soft" by scientists who are used to the laboratory setting. Such methods are being developed, with strong input from the social sciences and tailoring by clinicians (Deyo, 1984), and the case for their validity strengthened by evidence of content, construct, and criterion validity.

NEGATIVE TRIALS

Primary care physicians deal with diseases that have many causes, no single one of which may be much more powerful than the others. It is therefore not surprising for RCTs in this setting to demonstrate only small effects, or perhaps none at all, in studies of a single intervention. This can be a disappointment, because of our cultural bias in favor of positive findings, and so researchers are less likely to submit such studies for publication and journals less likely to publish them. But a negative trial of an important question can be just as useful as a positive one (Fletcher & Fletcher, 1986), if it shows that a common treatment is not effective or that a more expensive treatment is no more effective than a cheaper one.

There are two ways to deal with negative trials: to try to prevent them, and to make the most of the information they do contain. To prevent negative trials, they should be done meticulously. One is less likely to end up with a conclusion of "no difference" when there truly is one if the effect is not obscured by error attributable to faulty measurements, low compliance, cointerventions, and the like. When trials are planned, there should be good reasons, both theoretical and from data-based research, for believing that an intervention is promising before going to the effort of studying it in a randomized trial. It may be prudent to study the effects of a set of interventions, selected to have the largest expected effect, rather than only one: If the aggregate is effective, one can then go on to do more targeted studies to find out which component made the difference. If a set of interventions is not effective, it is unlikely that the individual components are. Either way, there is an answer. Finally, one can reduce the chances of a false negative study by enrolling an adequate number of patients in the trial. If resources are limited but patients are not, it may be best to gather fewer variables on many patients rather than many variables on few. If patients are in short supply, a multicenter study may be necessary.

To get the most information out of a study, whether its findings are negative or positive, the main measure of effect for the trial should be summarized as a "point estimate" (the actual size of the treatment effect observed in the study) and a confidence interval (Gardner & Altman, 1989). This practice is recommended by most major journals (Bulpitt, 1987; Rothman, 1979). It gives both researchers and readers the most likely effect, based on the study, and the range of values that is likely to include the true one. Probability values ("p-values") obscure this information by pulling emphasis away from the size of the treatment effect and by including an arbitrary value judgment about what is or is not likely to have occurred by chance.

If the results of a trial are consistent with a wide range of effect sizes, some large and others very small, the study does not advance our understanding much. Therefore, we need to plan studies that end with a useful degree of precision for the main effects—that is, where one can be reasonably certain that the true effect of the intervention is within a relatively narrow range of values. This is accomplished by studying a large number of patients; obtaining a high rate of outcome events in those who are studied; and by reducing the variation in the sample by restrictive entry criteria, matching, or modeling.

When confidence intervals are presented, the researchers—and, for that matter, the readers—are empowered; they can hold their own opinions about what is a clinically important effect size up to the confidence interval to see if it is included. For example, if a trial shows that the effectiveness of a new treatment on plantar wart regression is unlikely to be more than 5%, then most readers would consider this a negative trial; even the biggest plausible effect is still too small to be clinically important. In contrast, if the 95% confidence interval for relative risk of sudden death during exercise is 10-150, even the lowest plausible risk is still large, although we have little precision on just what the risk is (Siscovick, Weiss, Fletcher, & Lasky, 1984).

UNIT OF ANALYSIS

The unit of analysis may not be the same as the unit of randomization. For example, one may randomize physicians but measure outcomes on their patients, or randomize clinics but study the effects on physicians' practices. This situation seems to arise more often in studies of primary care than in more biomedically oriented settings. (In Dr. Labrecque's study, reported in Chapter 5, patients were randomized and, quite appropriately, patients rather than their warts were considered the unit of analysis.)

Primary care researchers should be aware that the unit of analysis is not necessarily a straightforward issue and could affect both the determination of adequate sample size when the study is being planned and the appropriate form of analysis after the data are collected. Unit of analysis is a problem mainly if it is not recognized and given sufficient attention; biostatisticians and other methodologists can help with the decisions that must be made.

Conclusions

Clinical trials of primary care interventions are in their infancy. If they are done well, they can have far-reaching consequences. This is a wonderfully exciting time to be in such a field, at the beginning of what might be a rapid growth phase, where much is at stake and nothing yet assumed. To meet the challenges and to fulfill their potential, primary care researchers will have to depart from their current paradigms. Some will need to get advanced training in clinical research methods; all will need to give up some of their clinical freedom—and persuade their patients to do the same—to participate in trials. They will need to work with specialists in research design as well as in analysis—scholars who may not have been part of their working group before. They will need to submit themselves to the rigors of external review, to obtain grants, and to publish papers—and the reviewers will not necessarily be sympathetic to primary care. The end result of such efforts could be a new level of effectiveness in primary care.

This chapter has provided a theoretical overview of RCTs in primary care. But theory is only a prelude to action, which in research means actual design, measurement, and analysis of data bearing on an important question. The following chapters illustrate some of the concepts I have introduced with actual examples.

References

Anonymous. (1980). Opie and the heart. *Lancet, 1,* 692.

Braitman, L. E. (1991). Confidence intervals assess both clinical significance and statistical significance. *Annals of Internal Medicine, 114*(6), 515-517.

Bulpitt, C. J. (1987). Confidence intervals. *Lancet, 1,* 494-497.

Deyo, R. A. (1984). Measuring functional outcomes in therapeutic trials of chronic disease. *Controlled Clinical Trials, 5,* 223-240.

Feinstein, A. R. (1983). An additional basic science for clinical medicine: II. The limitations of randomized trials. *Annals of Internal Medicine, 99,* 544-550.

Fletcher, R. H. (1990). Three ways of knowing in clinical medicine. *Southern Medical Journal, 83,* 308-312.

Fletcher, R. H., & Fletcher, S. W. (1986). Negative trials. *Journal of General Internal Medicine, 2,* 285-287.

Fletcher, R. H., Fletcher, S. W., & Wagner, E. H. (1988). *Clinical epidemiology: The essentials* (2nd ed.). Baltimore, MD: Williams and Wilkins.

Friedman, L. M., Furberg, C. D., & DeMets, D. L. (1985). *Fundamentals of clinical trials* (2nd ed.). Littleton, MA: PSG.

Gardner, M. J., & Altman, D. G. (1989). *Statistics with confidence: Confidence intervals and statistical guidelines.* London: British Medical Journal.

Pocock, S. J. (1983). *Clinical trials: A practical approach.* New York: John Wiley.

Rothman, K. (1979). A show of confidence. *New England Journal of Medicine, 299,* 1362-1363.

Sackett, D. L., Haynes, R. B., Guyett, G. H., & Tugwell, P. (1991). *Clinical epidemiology: A basic science for clinical medicine* (2nd ed.). Boston: Little, Brown.

Siscovick, D. S., Weiss, N. S., Fletcher, R. H., & Lasky, T. (1984). The incidence of primary cardiac arrest during vigorous exercise. *New England Journal of Medicine, 311,* 874-877.

4 Evaluating the Effectiveness of a Multifaceted Community-Based Support Program

E. ANN MOHIDE

This chapter describes the evaluation of a multifaceted community-based support program to illustrate some of the design, measurement, and analysis issues raised by Dr. R. Fletcher in his overview of important theoretical aspects of trials in primary care (Chapter 3). The randomized trial reported here looked at family caregiver support for the home management of older people suffering from progressive irreversible dementia and provides examples of specific methodological issues. Such issues include the trade-off between generalizability and internal validity; the impossibility of blinding; adherence to treatment; contamination; cointervention; selection of a credible, feasible, reliable, and valid outcome measure; attrition; and the interpretation of negative results.

Study Background and Overview

The problems associated with caring for relatives suffering from progressive irreversible dementias have been demonstrated in numerous studies. At the time this study was designed, however, few investigations examining the impact of interventions on family caregivers had been reported, and none addressed the multidimensional nature of caregiver problems. These problems included the need for physical relief from caregiving; perceived health problems; deficits in caregiving knowledge, skills, and problem solving; and the need for self-help support networks. With these facts in mind, a randomized trial (Mohide et al., 1990) was conducted to determine the effectiveness of a set of supportive interventions in reducing burden on family caregivers managing moderately to severely demented elderly at home. Called the Caregiver Support Program (CSP), the study was funded over a 3-year period by the Ontario Ministry of Health, Research and Planning Division.

Caregiver-patient pairs ($N = 60$) were recruited from an urban center in southern Ontario and block-randomized to receive either the experimental CSP intervention, or conventional community nursing care, over a 6-month period. The CSP intervention consisted of caregiver-focused health care, education about dementia and caregiving, assistance with problem solving, regularly scheduled in-home respite, and a self-help caregiver support group. The conventional community care focused on care of the demented patient rather than on the caregiver. Nurses in that group did not have special training and did not recommend any of the above services in a standardized or systematic manner.

Methods

RATIONALE FOR THE DESIGN

Primary care interventions often need to be multidimensional in nature, a point amply illustrated here—the problems of family caregivers make it unlikely that any single intervention would result in a substantial effect. Based on this reasoning and on the fact that the sample size required for a factorial design was not attainable, a set of several individual interventions was evaluated. If the entire set could be shown to be effective, then further studies could be conducted to examine the relative effectiveness of the components.

The decision was made also to offer a form of treatment to the conventional care group, because subjects probably would not have agreed to be assigned to a "no treatment" alternative, especially those who were receiving some form of community care at the time of recruitment. Aside from the loss of potential subjects that this might have led to, it is unlikely that those who agreed to be randomly allocated to a "no treatment" group could have been maintained in this "natural" state. As primary care clinicians can attest, the biopsychosocial complications of progressive irreversible dementias inevitably bring the patient and/or caregiver into contact with the health care system, and in almost all cases this leads to the initiation of some form of intervention. Thus the comparison group would be lost. Some consideration was given to observing a group of caregivers in the community; however, preliminary sample size estimates indicated that the assembly of a third group of subjects bearing similar characteristics to those in the other two groups would not be possible.

SUBJECTS AND ELIGIBILITY

To be eligible for enrollment in the trial, both the caregiver and his or her cognitively impaired relative had to satisfy certain inclusion criteria that were set to increase homogeneity and thereby reduce the "noise" relative to the "signal." First, they had to live together: The role and types of problems would be expected to differ for caregivers living with the demented relative in comparison with those not in coresidence. Second, medically diagnosed confirmation of progressive irreversible dementia was required, to ensure the exclusion of patients suffering from disorders such as a reversible form of dementia, depression, or delirium. If such cases were included and caregivers were shown to improve over the course of the study, it would not be clear whether this improvement was a result of the intervention or of the improved status of the patient. Other criteria, such as the exclusion of patients with life-threatening disease or who were likely to be institutionalized during the intervention periods, were established to minimize attrition.

As Dr. Fletcher has pointed out, restrictions such as these are designed to increase the internal validity of the study, but they often diminish the generalizability of the findings, that is, the extent to which this study population is representative of the typical primary care situation. Many individuals face concomitant illness, uncertainty about long-term placement plans, or less than clear-cut diagnoses. Such restrictions were necessary, however, as not enough subjects were available to enable meaningful subgroup analyses. A multicenter trial would have increased the numbers but also would have been costly and administratively complex, and it would have been difficult to establish and maintain comparability of community services and trial interventions across different urban centers. (Having said this, the point should be made that, had effectiveness been demonstrated for our restricted sample, then the next step would have been to demonstrate effectiveness with relaxed sample specifications.) In an attempt to support the study's generalizability as much as possible to the "real world" of primary care, only about 10% of the subjects (unlike in many studies) were recruited and enrolled from tertiary care settings.

The eligibility procedures involved a number of labor-intensive sequential steps, although these were designed to maximize the efficiency of the research staff. All screening tests and batteries demonstrated adequate psychometric properties. A log of consecutive potential subjects was maintained. Basic characteristics and the reason for ineligibility were documented, thereby permitting the comparison of those who were enrolled with those who were not. Of 146 pairs assessed over a 6-month period, about 60% were found to be ineligible; a proportion that was relatively low for this type of study.

INTERVENTION ISSUES

To qualify as a "real-world" possibility for primary care, an intervention should be amenable to application in most communities and should not require the development of a new type of health professional or highly specialized service agency. Accordingly, community services were sought from existing agencies. Nursing services were obtained from the Hamilton-Wentworth and Halton Branches of the Victorian Order of Nurses (VON) Visiting Nursing Program, a nonprofit organization. "Respite workers" were recruited from another existing community agency, the Hamilton-Wentworth Visiting Homemakers Association.

To compensate for the fact that blinding of the study subjects was impossible, the group assignment was not identified to the subject as "experimental" or "conventional"; rather, the services to be provided in each group were described. Second, the research assistants instructed the subjects not to divulge the intervention(s) received. Finally, the principal investigator was blinded to the study adjudication, subject allocation, and operational issues with the clinical agencies.

The prevention, minimization, and/or assessment of biases resulting from cointervention and contamination required methodological consideration. To participate in the study, nurses had to not be contemplating a job change and had to have a minimum of one year of community nursing experience. Eleven volunteered; of these, three were randomly assigned to the experimental CSP intervention and the other eight to the conventional care group. The larger number of nurses providing care to the control group decreased the likelihood that they would change their practice because of the relatively large number of demented patients in their caseloads. If the nurses then provided more comprehensive care than expected, this change would be a cointervention; however, if they attempted to develop a set of interventions like the experimental set, *this* change would constitute contamination.

None of the nurses was permitted to provide services to subjects in the group other than the one to which they were assigned, and the CSP nurses were instructed not to talk about the interventions beyond their CSP peers and specially assigned supervisor. Finally, the scope of the data collection permitted the assessment of referrals and service patterns by study group (Drummond et al., 1991). While this would not prevent or minimize the possibility of cointervention or contamination, at least the extent to which these two biases might have been operating could be assessed.

MEASUREMENT

As is frequently the case in primary care research, the outcome of interest in this trial could not be measured directly as a physical finding or with a laboratory result, meaning that it would be classified as "soft." Ideally, the primary outcome variable would have been measurement of caregiver burden. The psychometric properties of several caregiver burden measures were appraised but, unfortunately, however, none of them had been shown to be responsive to change in previous intervention studies. Further, the development and validation of a new instrument measuring caregiver burden would require considerable time and research funds. Thus use of this type of measure was ruled out.

After ruling out caregiver burden measures, symptom-specific instruments that would reflect burden were examined. Because negative emotional affects, in particular depressive and anxiety symptomatology, were cited frequently in the literature, these were used as the major outcomes of interest. Measures with sound psychometric properties were selected: the Center for Epidemiologic Studies Depression Scale (CES-D; Radloff, 1977) and the state-anxiety portion of the State-Trait Anxiety Inventory (STAI; Spielberger, Gorsuch, & Lushene, 1968). Both of these measures have been shown to be reliable, valid, responsive to change, and feasible to use. Although they were not specific to the issues confronting caregivers, they permit comparisons with noncaregiving groups in the population. In addition, both instruments have been administered to samples from the general population, not just "sick" individuals. Of the two outcome measures, depressive symptomatology was deemed to be the most important in terms of morbidity and quality of life.

SAMPLE SIZE CONSIDERATIONS

Prior to developing the full proposal, a feasibility study was conducted to determine the willingness of family physicians to participate in the study as well as to determine the number of patients in their practices who would meet the inclusion criteria. On the basis of this, it was estimated that it would be feasible to enroll a total of 65-70 subjects in the study over a 6-month period. An attrition rate of not more than 15% was expected, because a number of methodological strategies were to be incorporated to minimize dropouts (e.g., inclusion criteria and keeping the intervention period relatively short). Therefore, it was expected that roughly 28-30 subjects per group would complete the trial. With the standard deviation of 10 points on both the CES-D and STAI scales, and the Type I error (alpha) set at .05, this would yield slightly less than 80% power to detect a difference of 7 points in either scale between the experimental and the control groups, using a two-tailed test (Colton, 1974). This would amount to an effect size of 0.7, which, according to Cohen (1988), is large. Differences smaller than 7 points were not judged to be clinically significant.

Results

Sixty caregivers were enrolled in the trial, but only 42 (70%) completed it: 22 in the experimental and 20 in the control group. Almost all (89%) withdrawals were due to institutionalization of the demented relative. This high attrition rate occurred despite the relatively short intervention period and the precaution of screening out those who were not likely to remain at home.

Effectiveness analyses were conducted only on those subjects who completed the trial. The reasons were, first, that more data were available, and, second, the results did not differ from those obtained in an intention-to-treat analysis, which included those who completed at least 18 weeks of the intervention.

Caregivers suffered from depressive symptomatology and anxiety above the levels that would be expected for the general public but not in the moderate to high range. Neither group intervention reduced the levels of these, nor did the groups differ statistically. Examining these data using 95% confidence intervals, the largest plausible difference on the depressive symptomatology scale was not judged to be clinically important. With respect to the anxiety scale, the largest plausible difference might be judged to be clinically important (an 11-point difference); however, this finding is minimized by the lack of difference in depressive symptomatology, which is the more clinically relevant and important outcome.

Adherence to the study interventions, as in the real world, could not (and should not) be dictated. Although all experimental subjects accepted the three components delivered by the CSP nurse, 3 declined the in-home respite and 12 declined to participate in the support group. In the control group, one subject paid for respite services, and another independently joined a support group. Thus the potency of the experimental intervention may have been minimized because of rejection of some of its aspects and/or because the independent services obtained by the two control subjects might have minimized group differences.

One of the most important challenges to the implementation of a community-based health services protocol that may not be evident to the reader is the accurate estimation of the study personnel required to conduct a methodologically rigorous trial. In this study, the research component was demanding for the following reasons: (a) From referral to enrollment, the multistage sequential eligibility procedures required approximately 11.5 hours per caregiver-patient pair; (b) data collection was required from multiple sources: caregiver subjects, patients, physicians, nurses, and community agencies, including hospitals; (c) often multiple appointments were required to complete the interview schedules; (d) volunteers were needed in some cases to tend the demented relatives during interviews; and, finally, (e) the work load was increased substantially by the identification and measurement of all costs needed for a concurrent economic evaluation (Drummond et al., 1991). From the perspective of the clinical interventions under study, the coordination, training, and standardization of the interventions in the two community agencies were quite time-consuming. This work load included the development and implementation of two training programs, the establishment of a system of supervision for the clinical care, and the coordination of the research and clinical activities. Finally, each caregiver-patient pair required an assessment by a multidisciplinary clinical team upon trial completion or withdrawal, to ensure that adequate services were being substituted for those no longer available outside the study.

Conclusion

We identified the fact that these caregivers experience emotional symptomatology above the levels that would be expected for the general public. Neither intervention reduced these levels, however, nor did the groups differ statistically. Given the limited impact of this and other recently reported trials, a caregiver-focused intervention cannot be recommended at this point.

References

Cohen, J. (1988). *Statistical power for the behavioral sciences* (2nd ed.). Hillsdale, NJ: Lawrence Erlbaum.

Colton, T. (1974). *Statistics in medicine*. Boston: Little, Brown.

Drummond, M. F., Mohide, E. A., Tew, M., Streiner, D. L., Pringle, D. M., & Gilbert, J. R. (1991). Economic evaluation of a support program for caregivers of demented elderly. *International Journal of Technology Assessment in Health Care, 7*(2), 209-219.

Mohide, E. A., Pringle, D. M., Streiner, D. L., Gilbert, J. R., Muir, G., & Tew, M. (1990). A randomized trial of family caregiver support in the home management of dementia. *Journal of the American Geriatrics Society, 384,* 446-454.

Radloff, L. S. (1977). The CES-D Scale: A new self-report depression scale for research in the general population. *Applied Psychological Measurement, 1,* 385-401.

Spielberger, G., Gorsuch, R., & Lushene, R. (1968). *STAI manual for the State-Trait Anxiety Inventory.* Palo Alto, CA: Consulting Psychologists Press.

5 Evaluation of the Efficacy of a Homeopathic Treatment for Plantar Warts

MICHEL LABRECQUE

Planning and carrying out a "perfect" randomized controlled trial (RCT) for assessing an intervention in primary care is often a difficult if not impossible task. To illustrate both the methodological problems and the strengths associated with this research design, this chapter describes an RCT that evaluated the efficacy of a homeopathic treatment for plantar warts.

Methods

The research protocol was submitted to a homeopathic product company, which agreed to provide the medications and placebos as well as a grant covering the salary of a research assistant. The study was run at the Unité de Recherche Clinique en Médecine Familiale, a teaching family medicine unit at Laval University, Quebec. The medical staff of this unit comprises 12 full-time and 6 part-time family physicians and 24 family practice residents. The protocol was also accepted by the Ethics Committee of the Centre Hospitalier de l'Université Laval in Quebec City, Quebec, Canada.

SUBJECTS

The minimum number of subjects per group was calculated as follows. Based on the literature, we estimated that 50% of patients would have their warts disappear with the placebo treatment, and from this decided that 75% of our subjects should have healed warts for the treatment to be considered clinically effective. Finally, we set the α error (the p value) at 5% and the β error at 10%. Including an estimation of 15% loss to follow-up, this yielded a final recruitment goal of 200 subjects to end up with a minimum number of 85 per group (for a power of 90%).

In an attempt to maximize the homogeneity of the sample and thus the internal validity, inclusion in the study was originally restricted to patients between 6 and 29 years of age. Moreover, people with the following histories were excluded: previously treated warts, mosaic-type warts, a prescribed drug treatment for any condition, chronic disease, or immune deficiency. Pregnant or breast-feeding women and patients living outside the Quebec City area were also excluded, for ethical and practical reasons, respectively.

Patients were recruited from our own clinic as well as through local television, radio, newspapers, medical newsletters, and personal contacts with colleagues. We had hoped to recruit 10 patients per week over a 5-month period from December 1987 to May 1988; however, the process was slower than expected: Two weeks into the study, we had screened approximately 200 persons and recruited only 9! We then decided to be less restrictive on two eligibility criteria, extending the upper age limit to 59 years and including persons who had received treatment for their warts, as long as this treatment had occurred more than three months prior to entering the study. Despite these changes, we had to screen 853 persons over a 14-month period (December 1987 to January 1989) to enroll 174 subjects. Patients refused to participate ($n = 83$) or were excluded after completing a short questionnaire over the telephone ($n = 485$) or after a physical examination by a family physician ($n = 111$). Only the commitment of our research assistant, who offered to pursue her work on a quasi-voluntary basis when the funding ran out, enabled us to complete the study.

METHODOLOGICAL CONSIDERATIONS

1. Highly restrictive inclusion-exclusion criteria maximize homogeneity and hence internal validity but are a threat to both

generalizability and feasibility. Pretesting and close monitoring are essential to overcome this problem before it is too late, and it may sometimes be necessary to expand the criteria to preserve the feasibility of the trial.

2. A ratio of only one subject recruited out of five (or more!) patients screened is to be expected.

3. Surprises do occur. A dedicated and financially independent research assistant comes in handy.

PROCEDURE

Subjects were randomly allocated to receive either the homeopathic treatment ($n = 86$) or placebos ($n = 88$). Randomization was done by a hospital pharmacist who used a table of random numbers. The 6-week homeopathic treatment consisted of providing patients with three types of sugar pellets saturated with diluted tinctures, which they were to take sublingually at specified intervals. Treatments were dispensed in unit-dose tubes of approximately 200 micro pellets to be taken all at once or in tubes of 80 pellets. One contained Thuya 30CH, a tincture of cedar, diluted to 10^{-60} (one unit dose of 200 micro pellets once a week); one contained Antimony 7CH diluted to 10^{-14} (five pellets every day); and one contained nitric acid 7CH (one unit dose every day). Patients in the placebo group received pellets that looked and tasted exactly the same. As the treatment pellets were not expected to produce any side effects, complete blinding was achieved.

Over the 6 weeks, the nurse contacted patients every 10 days both to ensure the best possible compliance with the treatment and to inquire about side effects. At the end of the treatment period, compliance was verified by counting remaining unit-dose tubes and pellets. A patient was considered compliant if 80% of the medication had been taken.

MEASUREMENTS

The feasibility of this study was dependent on the collaboration of the participating clinicians, both for the initial diagnosis of warts and for the evaluation of healing. All the 12 full-time family physicians of the hospital-based family medicine unit agreed to participate, providing each of them would see only a few extra patients, thereby only minimally disturbing their routine activities.

Because multiple observers can lead to misclassification bias, objective criteria for clinical assessment were set. The diagnosis of warts was based upon the presence of hyperkeratosis, the interruption of skin folds, and the presence of micro thrombi. A wart was considered to have disappeared when skin folds were restored at the site previously infected, and a patient—our unit of analysis— was considered healed when *all* his or her warts had disappeared. The criteria were discussed by all the members of the unit, and clinical examples were illustrated on slides during a formal pre-study training session.

To increase validity, the criteria for inclusion in the study were deliberately made very specific and, if they were strictly applied, the probability of including someone with a lesion that was not a plantar wart would be very low. Nevertheless, to increase the specificity even more, patients had to have the diagnosis confirmed independently by two physicians. The amount of healing that had taken place by 6, 12, and 18 weeks also had to be assessed independently by two physicians. If their outcome assessments were different, a third physician was consulted independently to break the tie. We encountered such a situation only 10 times during the trial (2.7% of a total of 370 clinical assessments).

Despite constant efforts by the research assistant to have all the patients comply with their follow-up visits, an increasing number of subjects at each visit did not present: 29 (16.7%) at 6 weeks, 50 (28.7%) at 12 weeks, and 77 (44.3%) at 18 weeks. For most of these patients, their own assessment of healing was obtained by a phone call from the nurse.

Another outcome measure, the rate of healing of the warts as observed by the patient at 18 weeks, was recorded for all subjects.

METHODOLOGICAL CONSIDERATIONS

1. Validity of clinical measurement can be enhanced by the use of objective criteria by trained evaluators and by having more than one independent assessment done on each patient.

2. The longer the observation period, the higher the risk of noncompliance with the study protocol and of subject loss from the

Table 5.1 Subject Characteristics

| | Study Groups | |
| | Homeopathy | Placebo |
Characteristics	%	%
< 20 years old	19.8	37.5
Female	62.8	67.0
Wart(s) < 1 year old	47.7	67.0
Single wart	41.9	43.2
Painful wart(s)	53.5	54.5
Compliance	98.0	95.4
No other treatment(s)	76.3	85.4
Outcome assessment by MDs		
6 weeks	88.1	81.6
12 weeks	72.0	77.4
18 weeks	57.5	62.2
Complete follow-up	93.0	93.2

study. Subjects must be motivated to respect the study contract; phone calls, gifts, and money may help to keep them in the study. Researchers should be prepared to follow and assess the "defectors" through alternate means.

3. The use of "softer" tools for outcome evaluation (self-assessment versus clinical examination) increases the probability of misclassification bias.

Results

GROUP COMPARABILITY

The subjects in both groups were comparable in terms of sex, number of warts, reports of pain, compliance, attendance to follow-up visits, and loss to follow-up (Table 5.1). A 93% follow-up rate was achieved in both groups over the 18-week study period. Some differences were found between the two groups. Subjects in the treatment group were older, had warts for a longer period of time, and were more likely to have used another form of treatment than those in the placebo group.

METHODOLOGICAL CONSIDERATIONS

1. Randomization is likely to generate comparable groups, thus minimizing the risk for confounding bias. Comparability of the groups must still, however, be verified, especially if the sample size is small.

2. Achieving high follow-up rates minimizes the possibility of bias.

OUTCOMES

At the end of the 6-week treatment period, there was almost no difference between the proportion of patients healed in the homeopathy group (4.8%) and the placebo group (4.6%): 0.2% (95% confidence limits, −6.2%, 6.5%). Healing was also almost identical at 12 weeks: 13.4% in the homeopathy group and 13.1% in the placebo group, a difference of only 0.3% (95% confidence limits, −10.0%, 10.6%). At 18 weeks, a nonsignificant difference in favor of the placebo group (24.4%) over the homeopathy group (20.0%) was observed: −4.4% (95% confidence limits, −17.2%, 8.4%).

The proportion of patient-perceived improvement at 18 weeks was slightly lower in the homeopathy group than in the placebo group: 27.5% versus 33.3%, a difference of −5.8% (95% confidence limits, −19.5%, 8.7%); this difference, however, lacked statistical significance. Minor side effects (stomach aches, loose stools, and pimples) occurred very rarely with two patients on homeopathy and four on placebo.

We performed further analyses of subgroups of patients according to various prognostic factors (stratified analysis). The results remained the same for all variables, except for some nonstatistically significant effects of modification associated with age.

METHODOLOGICAL CONSIDERATION

The more simple a statistical analysis, the more understandable it will be. Dissimilarities between the groups must first be analyzed by stratification (subgroup analyses) and then, if necessary, by adjustment in a mathematical model.

Conclusion

Our RCT results show that the homeopathic treatment studied is no better than a placebo in treating plantar warts. The validity of this conclusion is supported by the study's adherence to such important principles as blinded assessments, compliance to a standardized intervention, and validity of measurement tools for inclusion in the study and outcome assessment.

The purpose here has been to illustrate some of the problems one can encounter in carrying out RCT studies, such as difficulties in subject recruitment and poor compliance to follow-up visits, and to report how we dealt with them. Solving these in-process problems proved possible with minimum threat to the study validity.

6 Randomized Trials
for Assessing Interventions
in Primary Care: Discussion

ALLAN DONNER

Chapter 3 discussed the theory behind the use of randomized trials to assess primary care interventions, while Chapters 4 and 5 presented two examples of recent trials. These trials, conducted by Professor Mohide and Dr. Labrecque, respectively, illustrate very well the methodological issues that can arise in primary care research and that reflect many of the points raised by Dr. Fletcher. In this chapter, we discuss these points further and summarize some key issues.

The Nature of the Intervention

The experimental intervention in Professor Mohide's trial was a multidimensional support system aimed at helping caregivers enhance their sense of competence and achieve a sense of control. While this type of intervention is relevant to primary care, its evaluation creates methodological difficulties that are usually not found in the evaluation of medical treatments. These are as follows:

(1) The effectiveness of the intervention is to a large degree directly influenced by the subject's own attitudes, motivations, and commitment to the goals of the study. To this extent, the opportunity for non-

compliance in a trial such as Mohide's is therefore greater than in drug trials.

(2) If the intervention is shown to have a statistically and clinically significant effect, its multidimensional nature makes it difficult to detect which of its components are contributing to the effectiveness. As emphasized by Dr. Fletcher, primary care physicians are generalists by choice and training and so may find it artificial to evaluate the components of an intervention separately. One might argue that this does not matter provided the intervention is always offered as a "package," but failure to disentangle its components limits our ultimate understanding of what is effective and what is not.

(3) Blindness of either the subjects or the investigators as to which intervention was being administered was clearly impossible in the caregivers' trial. One possible consequence is that the caregivers assigned to the experimental group might feel "favored" by receiving the support system, while those in the control group might feel at a disadvantage for not receiving it. It is well known that knowledge of the treatment group one is assigned to can directly affect the values of outcome measures, particularly when these measures are relatively "soft." A related issue is that the nurses' awareness of their group assignment might also have affected their management style in a way that is not reflective of real-life practice. This may be thought of as a placebo effect that falls upon the provider of health care rather than upon the patient. Unfortunately, these difficulties are largely unavoidable and suggest that, where possible, at least some outcome measures should be adopted that are relatively "hard" or objective. As Dr. Fletcher points out, however, it is often the relatively soft or indirect outcomes that are regarded as the most important in primary care, including psychological and social outcomes.

The Nature of the Control Group

In the plantar wart trial, the choice of a placebo control group was relatively straightforward. In the caregiver trial, however— as in many trials of the evaluation of multidimensional support systems—the choice was not as clear-cut. This is because, while a "no care" alternative was not considered feasible, there was also no established method of intervention that clearly defined a "standard care" group. The control group intervention that was ultimately selected by the investigators was conventional nursing treatment, which focused on the care of the demented relative rather than on the caregiver. But, as acknowledged by the investigators, conventional nursing care still contains elements of the experimental intervention, even though these elements are not its main focus. The effect of this is to dilute the differences between the treatment and control groups, thereby reducing the underlying statistical power of the trial. This type of cointervention is fairly typical of family medicine trials evaluating the effects of caregiving, where placebo controls are usually unethical or unfeasible.

It is also well known that the "social support," "attention," or other nonspecific components of such interventions may well be as important as the more specifically delineated medical and/or educational components. As Dr. Fletcher points out, these nonspecific effects are a vital part of the armamentarium of primary care physicians. One method of addressing this issue in the caregiver study might have been to have a second control group that was similar to the first except that it would explicitly provide social support to the caregivers as well as conventional nursing care to the patients. The resulting three-group design would help answer the question of whether it was the specific or nonspecific components of the intervention that were most effective. The disadvantages of this design are that it would add further administrative complexities and a larger required sample size to an already challenging enterprise. (For a discussion of issues involved in the choice of a control group in health care research, see Buck & Donner, 1982.)

The Nature of the Trial Setting

The trials reported by Labrecque and Mohide are both community based. Although such trials might be expected to have greater external validity than hospital-based ones, the difficulty, cost, and speed of recruitment are typically much greater than in the latter setting, where subjects are essentially "captive." Compounded by the need to adopt fairly strict inclusion/exclusion criteria, the time taken to enroll a suitable number of subjects may be inordinately great. As Fletcher and Labrecque both point out, the ratio of subjects recruited to those screened may be very small, and the resources needed to complete even the accrual stage of the trial are easily underestimated. One solution to this problem would be to broaden the inclusion/exclusion criteria. This would increase the generalizability of the trial results, but at the expense of diluting the effect of intervention and thus lowering the underlying statistical power. The difficulties in attaining a sufficient number of subjects have led Franks (1988) to suggest that only common problems should be addressed in family medicine trials. Fortunately, as pointed out by Dr. Fletcher, one advantage of randomized trials in a primary care setting is that relatively common conditions abound.

The opportunities for noncompliance are also greater in community-based trials. This is partly because there is simply greater difficulty in keeping subjects "on track" relative to hospital-based trials, where the opportunities for dropping out, missing appointments, and other forms of noncompliance are generally less frequent. This is reflected in the results reported by Dr. Labrecque, where the percentage of subjects presenting at each scheduled visit tapered off from about 85% at 6 weeks to only 60% at 18 weeks. When the intervention is largely under the control of the subject, as in the caregiver trial, problems of compliance can be even greater.

The Interpretation of a Nonsignificant Result

Both of the trials reported nonsignificant results for the comparisons of primary interest. As Professor Mohide acknowledges, the sample size in her trial was insufficient to detect clinically important differences between the groups on some key outcome variables. It is also made clear, however, that only a multicenter trial could have provided the required number of subjects, with all the associated difficulties of administrative complexity and protocol standardization. This dilemma—the ability to detect only very large treatment effects in single-center studies—is compounded by the fact that most primary care interventions are not likely to have hugely dramatic impact but to have effects that are small to moderate in size. This does not mean that they are not *important* to detect, given the large number of future patients who may benefit, simply that they are *difficult* to detect.

The use of confidence intervals to present major results in clinical trials is being increasingly encouraged (see Gardner & Altman, 1986). Confidence intervals summarize the uncertainty in an estimated intervention effect using a range of values, thus allowing the reader some flexibility in interpreting the trial findings. This is particularly important for nonsignificant trials, because it helps to place a reported lack of effect in proper perspective. A confidence interval of relatively narrow width is much more supportive of a negative result than is one whose limits encompass a broad range of possible values. Without a sample size sufficient to detect clinically important effects, however, the interpretation of a negative result in terms of "equivalence" is rarely justified. The determination of a sufficient sample size should be done on the basis of statistical power calculations, as discussed in many standard texts (e.g., Colton, 1974).

The Choice of Unit of Analysis

A characteristic of Dr. Labrecque's trial is that some patients contributed more than one wart to the analysis. Because it is possible to determine healing status separately for each wart, it is tempting to apply standard statistical methods to a combined sample of warts as obtained over all patients. This strategy can result in misleading conclusions, however, because responses on warts from the same patient are likely to be more similar than those on warts from different patients (i.e., to be positively correlated). The effect of within-patient correlation is to compromise the validity of standard statistical tests, resulting in p-values that are biased downward. The application of such procedures as t-tests or chi-square tests to a combined sample of observations obtained over all patients may well result in spurious statistical significance. One solution to this problem is to treat the *patient* as the unit of analysis, as in Labrecque's trial, where a "success" is defined as a patient whose warts have all healed. This is quite natural in the context of homeopathic treatment, because the focus of such treatment is on the patient rather than the site. There may be studies involving multiple sites per patient (e.g., warts, lesions, teeth), however, where the primary questions of interest would be more appropriately framed about the site rather than the patient; if this is the case, it is natural to retain the site as unit of analysis, while recognizing that relatively advanced statistical methods must be adopted to account for within-patient dependencies. For the case of continuous outcome measures, these methods, including repeated measures of analysis of variance, are fairly well established. For categorical outcome variables, however, the appropriate methods are still in the developmental stage, and the necessary computing software is not easily available.

Similar problems also arise when entire practices rather than patients are randomly assigned to interventions, a "group randomization" design increasingly adopted for a variety of practical reasons by primary care researchers. In this case, responses of patients within practices cannot be regarded as statistically independent, and the application of standard statistical methods to a combined sample of patient responses can again be misleading. For further discussion of this issue and additional examples, the reader is referred to Donner, Brown, and Brasher (1990) and Whiting-O'Keefe, Henke, and Simborg (1984).

Summary

The methodological issues involved in the evaluation of interventions in primary care are unique to the circumstances under which these evaluations are undertaken. The nature of the interventions, the nature of the trial setting, and the choice of unit of randomization may all be quite different than the usual clinical trial evaluation in which medical treatments are assigned to patients based in hospitals. This in turn affects how trials of primary care interventions should be designed and analyzed. The material presented in the last three chapters attempts to bring these distinctions out in the context of two recently completed intervention studies.

References

Buck, C., & Donner, A. (1982). The design of controlled experiments in the evaluation of nontherapeutic interventions. *Journal of Chronic Disease, 35*, 531-538.

Colton, T. (1974). *Statistics in medicine*. Boston: Little, Brown.

Donner, A., Brown, K. S., & Brasher, P. (1990). A methodological review of non-therapeutic intervention trials employing cluster randomization, 1979-1989. *International Journal of Epidemiology, 19*, 795-800.

Franks, P. (1988). Clinical trials. *Family Medicine, 20*, 443-448.

Gardner, M. J., & Altman, D. G. (1986). Confidence intervals rather than P values: Estimation rather than hypothesis testing. *British Medical Journal, 292*, 746-750.

Whiting-O'Keefe, Q. E., Henke, C., & Simborg, D. W. (1984). Choosing the correct unit of analysis in medical care experiments. *Medical Care, 22*, 1101-1114.

7 Theoretical Considerations of Qualitative Method: Behavioral Science Research of Relevance to Primary Care Interventions

JANIS H. JENKINS

This chapter selectively considers some of the theoretical foundations of qualitative research that are relevant to primary care interventions. Several fundamental questions can be posed: What is the nature of knowledge? Are there multiple forms of knowledge? How is it that we "know what we know"? What kinds of data count as evidence and meaningfully address our research questions? What analyses are usefully undertaken? How do we assess the validity of what we know? The assumptions that underlie each of these questions—that is, the theory of methodology—are inexorably part of the answers we might hazard. In my view, theory and method do not comfortably exist in isolation from one another; rather, theory dialectically implies method and method inherently reflects theory.

A Methodological Contrast: Qualitative Versus Quantitative Ways of Knowing

Competing epistemologies, or theories of the nature and grounds of knowledge, are what are at stake here. To consider the question: "What is qualitative knowledge and how is it presumed different than quantitative ways of knowing?" we turn to some remarks by Bogdan and Taylor (1975, p. 2) on the relationship of theory and method:

> Two major theoretical perspectives have dominated the social science scene. One, positivism . . . [considers] "social facts," or social phenomena, as "things" that exercise an external . . . influence on human behavior. The second theoretical perspective [is] described as *phenomenological*. . . . The phenomenologist is concerned with understanding human behavior from the actor's own frame of reference. . . . The phenomenologist examines how the world is experienced. For him or her the important reality is what people imagine it to be. Since the positivists and the phenomenologists approach different problems and seek different answers, their research will typically demand different methodologies. The positivist searches for "facts" and "causes" through methods such as surveys, questionnaires, inventories, and demographic analysis, which produce quantitative data and which allow him or her to statistically prove relationships between operationally defined variables. The phenomenologist, on the other hand, seeks understanding through such qualitative methods as participant observation, open-ended interviewing, and personal documents. These methods yield descriptive data which enable the phenomenologist to see the world as subjects see it.

Bogdan and Taylor do not say that positivists cannot employ qualitative methods to their own ends—qualitative data can certainly be used productively for causal or explanatory purposes. But researchers who collect such data are seldom searching for causes and explanations (Strauss & Corbin, 1990). More often, their goal is to understand the nature and meaning of human behavior.

Along with the substantive differences between the theoretical domains of quantitative and qualitative research strategies, there has long been an uneasy antagonism between the practitioners of these differing methods. As every reader knows, quantitative methods are very much the principal means of addressing the concerns of health care researchers today. Of course, qualitative biomedical types of knowledge do exist, but the dominant trend in health sciences research is the employment of positivist-empiricist approaches using quantitative methods. For example, the a priori assumption of the necessity for double-blind randomized controlled designs and large statistical data sets is widely shared. In primary care investigations, this is true for a wide set of research queries, from the identification of substrates of disease to the development and management of appropriate treatments.

Qualitative Methods and the Cultures of Medicine and Health Sciences Research

I would like to call attention to the bias that presumes that *quantitative* and *scientific* are synonymous terms, because recognition of this bias sheds light on the question of what counts as evidence and why. Preferences concerning the most valued types of data are central to an understanding of the "culture of medicine" (as Dr. Good terms it in Chapter 10) and are constitutive of fundamental presuppositions in scientific discourse on health, illness, and disease. By the *culture of medicine*, I mean the set of shared actions and meanings that pervade medical settings. The notion of culture employed here is that behaviors and attitudes are generally shared and taken for granted. Like other social settings, medical settings are inherently inscribed with core symbols and understandings of the way things are and should be. Indeed, strong sentiments are generally attached to these views.

To elaborate on the affective dimensions among various cultures of medicine and behavioral research in the health sciences, I draw on the notion of *ethos*, using this term in the way that anthropologist Gregory Bateson (1958) meant it when he introduced it in psychological anthropology more than three decades ago. Roughly, *ethos* refers to a standardized system of emotional attitudes. It can refer to the emotional environment of a whole culture, the communicative environment of a family, the consultation room in a primary care setting, or the meeting room for reviewers of scientific proposals submitted to the NIH.

The systematic pattern of emotional attitudes among cultural members constitutes the ethos of a particular group. In the context of health research today, the pervasive ethos surrounding qualitative research is to regard it symbolically as "soft," "fuzzy," "weak." Contrast, for example, the qualitative ethnographic approaches of anthropologists and the quantitative approaches that are the mainstay of epidemiology (Kleinman & Good, 1985, pp. 7-8):

Ethnography and epidemiological surveys sharply pose these differences. The former is qualitative and concerned principally with the problem of validity. [Epidemiology] is quantitative and concerned primarily with the problems of reliability and replicability. The ethnographer masters the local language, spends many months, even years, in the field, and develops close working relationships with a relatively small number of key informants. He or she concentrates on translation and interpretation of meaning. . . . The epidemiologist spends weeks, at most a few months, in the field, usually does not know the indigenous language and hence is forced to rely on questionnaires and measures of "observable" and "quantifiable" behavior. The epidemiologist views the ethnographer's task as "impressionistic," "anecdotal," "uncontrolled," "messy," "soft," "unrigorous," "unscientific"; the ethnographer, in near perfect counterpoint, regards the epidemiologist's work as "superficial," "biased," "pseudoscientific," "invalid," "unscholarly." Two unequal responses to this tension are apparent: the much more common—though to our minds less creative—is to put on blinders and disregard the work of the other; more rarely, researchers attempt to combine the two methods.

An example of how this integration has been made can be found in the work on anthropology and epidemiology by Janes, Stall, and Gifford (1986).

A feminist scholarly perspective would note that another bias to be acknowledged is the gender association often linked to quantitative and qualitative approaches (Farnham, 1987; Rosaldo & Lamphere, 1974), whereby the former is symbolically associated with male forms of knowledge and attributes, and the latter with female domains. Quantitative approaches are generally associated with "hard" data, randomized controlled design, and scientific objectivity and reliability; qualitative ones, with "soft" data, naturalistic techniques and uncontrolled design, and subjective impressionism and unreliability. The medical subdiscipline traditionally considered the "softest" of medical sciences—psychiatry—is commonly relegated a lesser prestige relative to subfields such as surgery or cardiology. One way in which academic psychiatry today has attempted to redress this "image problem" is to concentrate its energies more on studies of biological and anatomical markers, genetics, and psychopharmacology. While psychosocial investigation of major mental disorders is certainly still being pursued, it is increasingly becoming a less common endeavor.

A Qualitative Method Originating in Psychiatric Research

Some collaborative investigations that I have undertaken with colleagues have emphasized a blending of qualitative and quantitative approaches. Our research has concerned itself with the investigation of sociocultural factors and processes that mediate the course of psychiatric illness, especially schizophrenia and depression, and some of our conclusions have been used as the basis for subsequent family intervention studies (Jenkins, 1991; Jenkins & Karno, 1992; Jenkins, Kleinman, & Good, 1991; Karno et al., 1987). This work has specific applications to family medicine and primary care, as its methodologies and conceptual issues can also be usefully extended to studies of the course of a variety of potentially stress-related conditions or disorders, such as diabetes, hypertension, and asthma. This is so not only because primary care doctors are often the first (and sometimes the only) physicians to be consulted for diverse medical problems but also because the same basic psychocultural and behavioral processes may be at work for major depressive illness as for inflammatory bowel disease.

That sociocultural factors have proven important for the prognosis of even biogenetically regarded diseases such as schizophrenia invites research on a whole host of disorders that might similarly prove responsive to the social environment (Brown, Birley, & Wing, 1972; Jenkins & Karno, 1992; Karno et al., 1987; Vaughn & Leff, 1976a; Vaughn, Snyder, Jones, Freeman, & Falloon, 1984; WHO, 1979). One set of factors is the social and individual affective response to illness. For families, social response involves family attitudes and behaviors toward relatives with schizophrenia, such as protection, tolerance, criticism, or hostility (Jenkins, 1991). It is essential that illness and healing be examined within the most immediate of social contexts, that is, the family setting (Jenkins, 1988b; Kleinman, 1980). As patients' relatives will often vigorously and quite reasonably assert, systematic attention to family-based data constitutes a crucial source of information. I turn now to discussion of a particular qualitative-quantitative index of social response and support surrounding long-term illness: studies of "expressed emotion" as initiated in England by sociologist George Brown and his colleagues.

"Expressed emotion" (EE) is a research construct that provides a measure of criticism, hostility, and overinvolvement on the part of relatives toward an ill family member. Originally, the scope of EE research encompassed a much broader array of emotions and behaviors, but a specific focus on these three factors was adopted in light of numerous replication studies that demonstrated a statistically significant relationship between them and an exacerbation or clinical relapse of psychiatric symptoms (Brown et al., 1972; Karno et al., 1987; Leff et al., 1987; Vaughn & Leff, 1976a; Vaughn et al., 1984). The relationship between EE and clinical outcome in these studies has been found to be independent of clinical severity as measured by number of hospitalizations, length of illness, severity of symptomatology, and disturbed or highly aggressive symptom behaviors.

The beginning stages of EE research were exploratory. Researchers would visit family homes and qualitatively record ongoing behaviors and conduct interviews with key family members. This approach was intuitive-inductive and was designed to identify aspects of family interaction and relationships that might be important in pathways to recovery (Brown, 1985). Through open-ended questioning, the research interview, titled the Camberwell Family Interview (CFI), was developed over the course of several years. The interview is a semistructured questionnaire designed to elicit narrative accounts of everyday family life. Interviews are tape-recorded for subsequent analysis using the rating scales for EE. Training in the administration of the interview and reliable use of the rating scales generally take from 3 to 6 months. Vaughn and Leff (1976b) have more fully described the interview and rating scales elsewhere. (See Jenkins, 1991, for a review of how this method was cross-culturally adapted for use among Spanish-speaking families as well as a review of the qualitative coding of these interviews.)

In the past two decades, EE research has spread to five continents and has been extended to numerous disorders, psychiatric and nonpsychiatric alike (e.g., bipolar illnesses, dementia, anorexia nervosa, asthma, stroke, obesity, diabetes, and Parkinson's disease). While all this scientific activity might appear to signal advancement in a highly developed research paradigm, a major drawback of this work has been the lack of attention to its theoretical underpinnings. Cross-cultural analyses of this empirical index sheds light on this question (Jenkins & Karno, 1992). Through comparative analysis, it is evident that EE captures a broad-ranging set of essentially cultural factors in response to an illness, including conceptions of its nature and meaning, cultural rules for appropriate behavior and intimacy, and emotional styles within family contexts (Jenkins, 1988a, 1988b, 1991). To summarize, the principal value of EE research as a paradigm is that it serves (a) to identify major risk factors in the course and outcome of stress-related illnesses and (b) to offer a means for obtaining methodological rigor, reliability, and richness of psychocultural data.

Perspectives on the Nature of Communication and Implications for Doctor-Patient Interaction

Dr. Seifert (Chapter 9) asserts that "patients can teach *us* how to do research." I heartily endorse this premise and point here to three useful tools for examining it. Most fundamental is the well-known concept of "explanatory models" (EMs) introduced by Kleinman, Eisenberg, and Good (1978) more than a decade ago. EMs are views that patients, close family members, and physicians hold concerning the nature, cause, onset, pathophysiology, course, and preferred treatment for particular episodes of illness. Also included here are the emotional responses—often fear and anxiety—that surround an illness experience. It should come as no surprise that patients' and doctors' EMs are often quite different and sometimes in fact bear little relation to one another. EMs may be observed through naturally emerging discourse in the doctor-patient encounter or can be specifically elicited through a brief interview technique (Kleinman, 1980, p. 106).

Unfortunately, the idea that part of primary care practice should be to attend systematically to the patient's point of view appears to remain both novel and provocative. This neglect may be related in part to the relative valuation of different forms of knowledge on the part of physicians (biomedical and clinical over personal and familial) and in part to marked inequalities in the power relations between doctors and patients, whereby the latter are often embarrassed to impart their own views for fear of being ridiculed. The critical point is that considerably more than lip service must be paid to this idea in practice as well as in theory, because it is relevant not only to the task of immediate clinical care but also to the prediction of illness outcomes (Kleinman, 1988a).

A second useful tool is the "meaning-centered" approach developed in medical anthropology by Good and Good (1982, p. 147). This approach is distinct from the "disease-centered" empirical approach, which assumes the essential data are to be discovered and revealed. Instead, it focuses on the interpretation of language and behavior surrounding experiential illness realities.

The third tool endorsed here is narrative analysis: the recording of patients' and families' stories of experiencing illness. As observed by Kleinman in *The Illness Narratives* (1988b, p. 28):

> Symptom scales and survey questionnaires and behavioral checklists quantify functional impairment and disability rendering quality of life fungible. Yet about suffering, they are silent. The thinned-out image of patients and families that perforce must emerge from such research is scientifically replicable but ontologically invalid; it has statistical, not epistemological, significance; it is a dangerous distortion.

The narrative approach is also advocated by Miller and Crabtree (1990), who, in their article "Start with the Stories," called attention to the importance of everyday stories by patients and physicians for the questions these pose. These authors note that there are several different orders of knowledge embedded in the pressing questions encountered in everyday clinical encounters: (a) questions about *biology* such as blood pressure and cholesterol risk, natural history, and prognosis; (b) questions of *meaning*, such as "why me?" and "what is really known here?"; (c) *spiritual* questions of hope and despair, good and evil, emptiness, and sin; and (d) questions we would term *moral and emotional* responses to illness such as rage, vulnerability, pride and vanity, fear and insecurity, guilt and shame. The existential, spiritual, emotional, and moral meanings associated with illness are often considered within the realm of relatively devalued contexts—sometimes construed as misfortune, sometimes tragedy, and, as interpreted within North American popular psychology, within the realm of personal failure and defects of personality.

A somewhat different point concerns the multiple means through which this diverse set of questions is posed and responded to by patients and physicians. This involves inadequately understood forms of embodied knowledge that are less empirically observable but are nonetheless present in the form of a "sense" or "gut feeling." Qualitative methods are often meant to study these important sources of data, which fall into the category of the apparently unnameable "something" that so frequently informs clinical interactions. These are not the stuff of rationalist-empiricist quantitative approaches. Rather, they are the important grounds of intuitive bodily knowledge inherent in emotional atmosphere and bodily gestures that construct clinical communications and knowledge (Kestenbaum, 1982).

Concluding Comment

I conclude by summarizing principles common to qualitatively oriented researchers and primary care practitioners alike: (a) *holism*, the principle of interpreting and treating the patient within the context of his or her overall life experience; (b) *rapport*, the establishment of basic trust and communication between researcher and subject or doctor and patient that (implicitly or explicitly) offers support through nonjudgmental stances; (c) *empathy*, the willingness to engage actively in the patient's experience of illness and suffering; and (d) *intersubjectivity*, the interpersonally negotiated and interactively constructed affect-laden realities that are the very stuff of clinical encounters. Awareness of these basic principles can lead to empowerment in primary care interventions for patient and physician alike. Insistence upon a medical- or physician-based reality that is devoid of the patient's world contributes to the breakdown of those shared collaborations and meanings that are so essential to knowledge and healing.

References

Bateson, G. (1958). *Naven*. Stanford, CA: Stanford University Press.

Bogdan, R., & Taylor, S. J. (1975). *Introduction to qualitative research methods: A phenomenological approach to the social sciences*. New York: John Wiley.

Brown, G. (1985). The discovery of expressed emotion: Induction or deduction? In J. Leff & C. Vaughn (Eds.), *Expressed emotion in families*. New York: Guilford.

Brown, G., Birley, J. L., & Wing, J. (1972). Influence of family life on the course of schizophrenic disorders: A replication. *British Journal of Psychiatry, 121*, 241-258.

Farnham, C. (1987). *The impact of feminist research in the academy*. Bloomington: Indiana University Press.

Good, B., & Good, M. D. (1982). Toward a meaning centered analysis of popular illness categories. In A. Marsella & G. White (Eds.), *Cultural conceptions of mental health and therapy*. Dordrecht, Holland: D. Reidel.

Janes, C., Stall, R., & Gifford, S. (1986). *Anthropology and epidemiology*. Dordrecht, Holland: D. Reidel.

Jenkins, J. H. (1988a). Conceptions of schizophrenic illness as a problem of nerves: A comparative analysis of Mexican-Americans and Anglo-Americans. *Social Science and Medicine, 26*, 1233-1243.

Jenkins, J. H. (1988b). Ethnopsychiatric interpretations of schizophrenic illness: The problem of nervios within Mexican-American families. *Culture, Medicine, and Psychiatry, 12*, 303-331.

Jenkins, J. H. (1991). Anthropology, schizophrenia, and expressed emotion: The 1990 Stirling Award essay in ethos. *Journal of Psychological Anthropology, 19*(4), 387-431.

Jenkins, J. H., & Karno, M. (1992). The meaning of "expressed emotion": Theoretical issues raised by cross-cultural research. *American Journal of Psychiatry, 149*, 9-21.

Jenkins, J. H., Kleinman, A., & Good, B. (1991). Cross-cultural studies of depression. In A. Kleinman & J. Beckers (Eds.), *Psychosocial aspects of depression*. Hillsdale, NJ: Lawrence Erlbaum.

Karno, M., Jenkins, J. H., de la Selva, A., Santana, F., Telles, C., Lopez, S., & Mintz, J. (1987). Expressed emotion and schizophrenic outcome among Mexican-American families. *Journal of Nervous and Mental Disorders, 175*, 143-151.

Kestenbaum, V. (Ed.). (1982). *Humanity of the ill: Phenomenological perspectives*. Knoxville: University of Tennessee Press.

Kleinman, A. (1980). *Patients and healers in the context of culture*. Berkeley: University of California Press.

Kleinman, A. (1988a). *Rethinking psychiatry*. New York: Free Press.

Kleinman, A. (1988b). *The illness narratives: Suffering, healing, and the human condition*. New York: Basic Books.

Kleinman, A., Eisenberg, L., & Good, B. (1978). Culture, illness, and care. *Annals of Internal Medicine, 12*, 83-93.

Kleinman, A., & Good, B. (Eds.). (1985). *Culture and depression: Studies in the anthropology and cross-cultural psychiatry of affect and disorder*. Berkeley: University of California Press.

Leff, J., Wig, N., Ghosh, A., Bedi, H., Menon, D. K., Kuipers, L., Korten, A., Ernberg, G., Day, R., Sartorius, N., & Jablensky, A. (1987). Expressed emotion and schizophrenia in north India. III: Influence of relatives' expressed emotion on the course of schizophrenia in Chandigarh. *British Journal of Psychiatry, 151,* 166-173.

Miller, W. L., & Crabtree, B. F. (1990). Start with the stories. *Family Medicine Research Update, 9,* 2-3.

Rosaldo, M., & Lamphere, L. (1974). *Woman, culture, and society.* Stanford, CA: Stanford University Press.

Strauss, A., & Corbin, J. (1990). *Basics of qualitative research: Grounded theory, procedures, and techniques.* Newbury Park, CA: Sage.

Vaughn, C., & Leff, J. (1976a). The influence of family and social factors on the course of psychiatric illness: A comparison of schizophrenic and depressed neurotic patients. *British Journal of Psychiatry, 129,* 125-137.

Vaughn, C., & Leff, J. (1976b). The measurement of expressed emotion in the families of psychiatric patients. *British Journal of Social and Clinical Psychiatry, 15,* 157-165.

Vaughn, C., Snyder, K., Jones, S., Freeman, W. B., & Falloon, I. R. (1984). Family factors in schizophrenic relapse: Replication in California of British research on expressed emotion. *Archives of General Psychiatry, 41,* 1169-1177.

World Health Organization. (1979). *Schizophrenia: An international followup study.* New York: John Wiley.

8 Hearing a Word, Sensing What's Wrong, Finding a Way: Physicians' Responses to Patients' Concerns

DENNIS G. WILLMS

A life as lived is what actually happens. A life as experienced consists of the images, feelings, sentiments, desires, thoughts, and meanings known to the person whose life it is. One can never know directly what another individual is experiencing, although we all interpret clues and make inferences about the experiences of others. (Bruner, 1984, p. 7)

The life history that we wish to interpret is something whose meaning is revealed not by imposing external constructs but by "making room" to accommodate the foreign frame of reference that brought it into being. (Watson, 1976, p. 101)

One of the challenges of clinical medicine today is to balance professional explanation (the interpretive rules of science) with personal interpretation (the interpretive rules of common sense, culture, and the wisdom of human relations). Stated differently, clinical medicine requires one to defer to biomedical rules of evidence (an efficacious medicine) all the while responding in a caring way to the concerns, worries, and emotional needs of the patient (an effective medicine). To what extent, however, do clinicians trust the latter approach? And, if they do, how does it work? How is it done? Can they trust the hunches, intuitive skills, and personal interpretation that derive from their experience with patients?

Miller and Crabtree (1990, pp. 2-3) recognize this division in rules of evidence and in ways of knowing and believe that the two interpretive worlds can be bridged:

> Our research has been separated from the stories; our science has broken its covenant with *practice*. The clinician in us recognizes this brokenness and searches for alternatives to the traditional epidemiological research methods, such as *"qualitative"* approaches, but often returns home from this search uncertain, fearful, even angry. Why? (emphasis added)

Is this "brokenness" they referred to—between the "evidence-based medicine" of science and the "experience-based medicine" of practice—a product of this lack of trust? We can certainly trust science, but can we trust the human clues? It is not surprising that this distrust is doubly alienating. First, it generates professional insecurities ("Can I trust these hunches that I have about this patient?" "I should just stay with the clinical evidence, shouldn't I?"). Second, by not responding to their personal hunches, physicians personally alienate themselves from their patients ("My doctor doesn't really understand what's going on . . . what my real problems are"). I argue, as do Miller and Crabtree, that convergence is possible. This chapter concentrates on that part of the clinical moment where personal interpretation is most evident.

Miller and Crabtree (1990, p. 2) challenge physicians to start with the "stories" to enter into the patient's world of concern and worry, hopes and fears, dilemmas and misgivings. Yet who has the time? Is there time to listen to the whole story, the patient's version of the truth? Perhaps, for family practice physicians, who get to know patients and their families over time, these stories can unfold; short excerpts that, strung together, paint the larger picture. But when time is at a premium, are words enough?

In every culture, certain words have come to suggest, even represent, a particular kind of story. Whether it is *heart distress* in Iran (Good, 1977) or *nerves* in Newfoundland (Davis & Guarnaccia, 1989), these words—emotionally charged, socially and culturally loaded—flesh out a predictable set of human circumstances. I argue in this chapter that, by "listening to the words," words that in themselves are glimpses of the whole story, the physician can often sense what's wrong; by responding with care, he or she may then find a more compelling way to ameliorate patient concerns.

This chapter describes how a qualitative study of heavy smokers caused us to reconsider the structure and content of a smoking cessation intervention. The stories of these persons—as to how and why they smoked and their experiences of attempting to quit— provided a rich and detailed account of the struggles, tensions, worries, and dilemmas of everyday life. Smoking was a symptom of their troubles; a reflection of discontent. Some of their stories were contained in a key word; often, the words would be the same across different people because the problem was a reflection of similar experiences.

Background to the Qualitative Study

The qualitative study that generated these observations came about as a side study to a larger clinical trial. The primary research objective of the main study was to evaluate the effectiveness of a clinical maneuver that family practice physicians could use in helping their patients stop smoking: specifically, providing them with a nicotine-bearing chewing gum, Nicorette (Gilbert et al., 1989; Lindsay et al., 1989; Wilson et al., 1988). Physicians in the experimental condition were given a 4-hour, continuing medical education workshop designed to teach them the highly structured smoking cessation protocol used with the gum. The clinical assumption for this intervention was predicated on pharmacophysiological and behavioral principles: Persons smoke because of (a) their dependence on nicotine (addiction models) and (b) frequently repeated habits (behavioral models).

In our group of researchers, a multidisciplinary team of clinicians, biostatisticians, health educators, social scientists, and clinical psychologists, it was felt that these existing explanations were insufficient. Cigarette smoking, we felt, is a complex behavior influenced by a wide range of biological, psychological, and sociocultural factors; yet little is known about *why* or *how* persons smoke or, for that matter, the "stages and problems associated with cessation" (Best, 1983). Furthermore, because smoking behavior is socially and culturally constructed, appropriate understandings of its experiences and processes should reflect not only biological and behavioral perspectives but social and cultural ones as well.

Design of the Qualitative Study

The objectives of the qualitative research study were twofold: (a) to examine the social-cultural determinants of smoking and (b) to understand more fully the complex factors that influence cessation processes.

To that end, five family practice physicians in southern Ontario invited patients who were heavy or habitual smokers (20 or more cigarettes per day) to participate in this study. Participants (a) had to consent to try to quit smoking with the help of their physician and (b) had to agree to be interviewed subsequently at least 11 times over the next year. The first interview was scheduled shortly after the recruitment visit; subsequent interviews were scheduled once a month following the patient's quit day.

We recruited 43 subjects for the study. Interviews were conducted by a research assistant trained in qualitative research methods and were held in the participants' homes or occasionally at their workplaces. An open-ended, relatively unstructured interviewing method was used (see Agar, 1980), and interviews were audiotaped and transcribed for later analysis. We relied heavily on language, scrutinizing the words that the patients used to communicate their experiences in smoking and in attempting to quit. That is, the language of smoking—either literally or, in the context of a story, metaphorically—provided our data base.

We constructed four steps for our analysis and interpretation of the qualitative material: (a) interviews and field notes, (b) case studies, (c) codes—the problems, issues, and themes that derived from the texts—and (d) emergent theory—the constructs, idioms, and typologies of smoking experience and cessation (see Willms et al., 1990). That is, over the year of interviews that constituted stage 1, a story unfolded for each participant that reflected his or her concerns, troubles, and worries in attempting to quit or successes in quitting. In the second stage of the analysis, these experiences were turned into individual case studies (stories), which were then content-analyzed, compared with other stories, and developed into representations of smoking experience. Often, a single word or metaphor would capture the essence of a person's story.

This chapter concentrates on the second stage of interpretation: the case study or story. One of these stories, that of "Karen" is representative.

KAREN'S STORY

Karen's experience as a smoker—with a period of 9 months as a successful quitter—is an interesting example of the correlation between feeling "settled" or secure (in relationships, finances, and self-identity) and the ability to quit smoking. At those times in her life when she felt "stuck" (unsettled, caught in her situation at home), she spoke of being frequently depressed and of the need to smoke. Stated another way, when she saw herself as an individual—confident, secure, and independent—there was no need for her to smoke (Willms, 1991). This independence was, she felt, sustained by a supportive family, life-style options that were not previously available (e.g., exercise classes, "time-out" with friends), and a growing perception that she was "in control" of her life. Yet, when these perceived securities were undermined or taken away, she intentionally resumed smoking. In response to her physician's frequent challenges to quit, she would give responses such as, "How can I when I'm stuck at home?" or "I need them for my nerves!" Months later, feeling "in control," she was ready and able to quit. Here is her story:

At the time of our study, Karen was a 30-year-old woman who had been married for 12 years. She has two sons and works as a homemaker. For 8 years prior to the birth of her first child, she held a job outside of the home. She said that becoming a housewife was somewhat of a "culture shock." She felt "stuck," confined, and she suffered from a "lack of stimulus" (see Figure 8.1). She had a "tendency toward depression," and her physician, hearing these words, told her that her problems were psychosomatic. At the time of my interviews with her, Karen felt that her life was getting better. Her children were now older, her husband's job was more secure, and she saw her "own emergence as an individual again."

Karen had starting smoking in her teens as a means of rebelling against her parents and to be a part of the "in crowd" (see Figure 8.1). A few years later, she was doing it for other reasons: It made her feel "glamorous." When she became a mother, smoking was the social thing to do with other women—sitting around with coffee, the kids crying, and smoking. Karen said that, every year or so, she would talk about quitting; however, as soon as she cut down on her cigarettes, her weight would go up 2 or 3 pounds. At the age of 24, realizing that she had smoked for nearly half her life, Karen quit "cold turkey." She started again 6 months later, after she had gained 25 pounds.

Karen felt that she was "emotionally" rather than "physically" addicted to cigarettes, for her smoking was more "socially related." Cigarettes gave her "a way of feeling comfortable" and something to do with her hands in social situations. She and her husband were invited to a lot of business dinners; smoking allowed her to feel more comfortable on these occasions. Quite often, she would smoke an entire package in one evening and come home feeling terrible.

Her decision to quit was predicated on feeling that she was "more in control" than ever. She was "free" to do many of the things she had wanted to do for years: play tennis, get out of the house from time to time with her friends, and "be herself." Her husband's business was more successful than ever, and he too was independent of his father, the president of the company. She was ready to try to quit smoking, and her husband supported her all the way. He even stayed home from work on her first day of quitting, to "protect me from the kids, and the kids from me."

At one of her first social engagements after quitting, Karen explained to her friends that she was attempting to stop smoking ("If I act strange, that's why!"). She made it through this first experience with relative ease, but about a month later a business convention in Quebec proved more difficult. Many of the women she socialized with were smoking; cigarette packages littered the tables. She felt like "Mrs. In-Between." That is, she did not consider herself a "nonsmoker" yet, and the nonsmokers present had no sympathy for her because they did not know what she was going through—but she didn't fit in with the smoking group either, as her presence put them on the defensive. She felt that they were

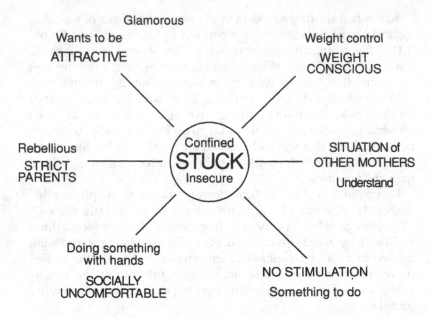

Figure 8.1. Multiple Meanings of Key Word *Stuck* and How Smoking
Functions to Address the Many Problems Associated with
Being "Stuck"

treating her "like the plague" because she was doing something
they wished they could do (see Figure 8.2). Despite these feelings,
she persevered.

It was at another business convention in New Orleans, however,
that she "threw in the towel." Her relapse, she said, was a reaction
to the behavior of her husband. He was flirting with a waitress and
she felt threatened and angry. She told me that she started smoking
again to "get back at him." It was the thing that he hated most about
her: "my smoking."

Discussion

This qualitative study made us reexamine our assumptions
about why it is that people smoke. They smoke because they are
addicted to nicotine and because they are behaviorially dependent,

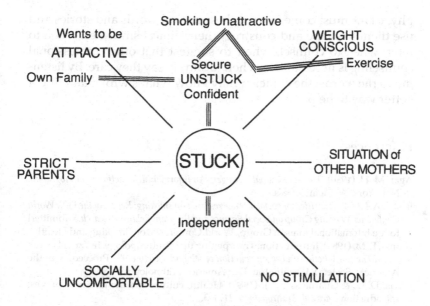

Figure 8.2. The Shift from Being "Stuck" to Being "Unstuck": An
Emerging Pattern of Confident Living

but also, and more important for some, for social reasons. These
reasons—expressed in words that tell a story (see Tambiah, 1968)—
are often more compelling and controlling of the smoking than is
the behavior or the addiction. Released from the constraints of
home, work, and troubling relationships, people may be ready and
able to quit. Karen's story is one example of many that provided
evidence of this.

For our group of coinvestigators, the qualitative results described above were used in the development of a more personal
and socially relevant smoking cessation intervention for clinical
practice (see Lindsay et al., 1989). Certain words—like "stuck,"
"weight," "nerves," "support," "worry"—would prompt use of
one strategy over another in challenging the patient to quit. Every
day, family practitioners hear such "platform words" (M. Seifert,
personal communication, 1991). These words give them something
to stand on, a place to start. They can lead to hunches or intu-
itions, thereby painting a kind of picture or profile of what problems a particular patient is experiencing. To intervene effectively,

physicians must come to trust these critical words and stories and use them to shape and construct their clinical strategies: when to refer, when to counsel, when to suggest that other professional counseling is necessary, or when to simply say they care. By listening to the words, the clinician may know what's wrong and find a better way to help.

References

Agar, M. H. (1980). *The professional stranger: An informal introduction to ethnography.* New York: Academic Press.

Best, J. A. (1983). *Priorities for social science research on smoking: Report of the Fifth World Conference Working Group on Social Science and Program Related Research.* Submitted to the International Liaison Group, World Conference on Smoking and Health.

Bruner, E. M. (1984). Introduction: The opening up of anthropology. In *Text, play, and story: The construction and reconstruction of self and society* (1983 Proceeding of the American Society). Washington, DC: American Ethnological Society.

Davis, D. L., & Guarnaccia, P. J. (1989). Health, culture and the nature of nerves: Introduction. *Medical Anthropology, 11,* 1-3.

Gilbert, J. R., Wilson, D. M., Best, J. A., Taylor, D. W., Lindsay, E. A., Singer, J., & Willms, D. G. (1989). Smoking cessation in primary care: A randomized controlled trial of nicotine-bearing chewing gum. *Journal of Family Practice, 28*(1), 1-7.

Good, B. (1977). The heart of what's the matter: The semantics of illness in Iran. *Culture, Medicine and Psychiatry, 1,* 25-58.

Lindsay, E. A., Wilson, D. M. C., Best, J. A., Willms, D. G., Singer, J., Gilbert, J. R., & Taylor, D. W. (1989). A randomized trial of physician training for smoking cessation. *American Journal of Health Promotion, 3*(3), 1-8.

Miller, W. L., & Crabtree, B. F. (1990). Start with the stories. *Family Medicine Research Update, 9*(2), 2-3.

Tambiah, S. J. (1968). The magical power of words. *Man (N.S.) 3,* 175-208.

Watson, L. C. (1976). Understanding a life history as a subjective document: Hermeneutical and phenomenological perspectives. *Ethos, 4,* 95-131.

Willms, D. G. (1991). A new stage, a new life: Individual success in quitting smoking. *Social Science and Medicine, 33*(12), 1365-1371.

Willms, D. G., Best, J. A., Taylor, D. W., Gilbert, J. R., Wilson, D. M. C., Lindsay, E. A., & Singer, J. (1990). A systematic approach for using qualitative methods in primary prevention research. *Medical Anthropology Quarterly, 4*(4), 391-409.

Wilson, D. M., Taylor, D. W., Gilbert, J. R., Best, J. A., Lindsay, E. A., Willms, D. G., & Singer. J. (1988). A randomized trial of a family physician intervention for smoking cessation. *Journal of the American Medical Association, 260*(11), 1570-1574.

9 Qualitative Designs for Assessing Interventions in Primary Care: Examples from Medical Practice

MILTON H. SEIFERT, JR.

The promise of practice research integrated with patient care has not become a practical reality. There are too few true collaborations and too little research on our basic beliefs. Our patients have no meaningful involvement in the process, except as subjects, and family practitioners are hardly ever involved in research design. There is not a consensus definition of quality of care, much less a means to measure quality.

We are concerned that researchers have overlooked the value of the practitioner and the patient as collaborators and the community practice as an empowering laboratory. This chapter provides examples to illustrate this value and to explain how it can become a reality.

Background Issues

THE PROMISE OF FAMILY PRACTICE RESEARCH

Some 20 years ago, family practice became a specialty, and it had some very high ideals. It would become a part of the university community and the medical center, and would participate in

---

AUTHOR'S NOTE: I wish to recognize the assistance of Mary Jo Good, Janis Jenkins, Benjamin Crabtree, and William Miller in the preparation of this chapter.

ongoing scholarly activities. Its main purpose would always be to promote a high quality of medical care, meaning care that was comprehensive and continuing, coordinated and accountable, and individualized to patients and their families.

Research would be done that would truly examine basic premises and core beliefs, with both academic and community practitioners collaborating throughout the research process, using the university as the core laboratory and the community settings as collaborating laboratory practices. In this idealistic view, the research agenda would focus first and foremost on quality improvement of health care services. It was expected that research efforts would be structured along the lines of ideal health care services; namely, collaborative, integrated, and coordinated. Both quantitative and qualitative research methods would be applied at the exploratory, descriptive, and explanatory phases with qualitative research holding the special promise of getting at what we saw and felt as clinical practitioners.

THE NATURE AND THE PROMISE OF QUALITATIVE RESEARCH

Qualitative research entails extensive fieldwork to describe and understand a culture. It uses participant observation and narrative accounts of human experiences in an effort to discover reality as it is; it expresses emotion, describes contexts, and discerns meanings. It can be used to describe and explain models of health care, to assess patient acceptance, and to evaluate patient satisfaction. Some would say it is well suited to primary care, and some would contend that it *is* primary care. These issues are, in fact, very close to the everyday reality of family practice physicians. The special promise of qualitative research is that it enables us to examine the core of our specialty to see who we are and what we do.

Qualitative research and primary care share many characteristics. The methods of each can be "low tech," but it is a mistake to think of these as less able to deal with complex issues. In fact, it is often the synergy of primary care and qualitative research that provides the means by which research becomes health care.

In this practitioner's view, a quality research design for assessing an intervention is one that improves the intervention as well as assessing it. This view sees the research process and the process of care as one. It also sees the physician as a researcher, the patient as a coresearcher, and the practice as a laboratory setting. The best design is the one that improves the efficiency of both practitioner and patient.

Unfortunately, although qualitative research is well suited to primary care, it is hardly ever used in practice settings in an *intentional* way. Rather, it is often seen as something apart from the care function. Neither physicians nor patients are trained in the use of qualitative methods, and practice sites are not thought of as places in which to do research.

Examples

The following are some examples of the use of focus groups to assess interventions in a community practice. The doctor and patient are seen as coresearchers and as focusing together on the process of care and how to improve it.

PATIENTS TEST AN ALREADY
TESTED DESIGN

Patients at our medical practice completed the Short Form 36 (SF36) as developed by John Ware et al. (see Stewart, Hays, & Ware, 1982; Wetzler, 1990) of the New England Medical Center. This instrument contains a number of separate scales that measure health status, social functioning, role functioning, mental health, pain, and energy level. Patients were asked to respond to the accuracy and usefulness of this information about themselves, as measured by the outcomes of their own testing. This took place in the context of a focus group at a regular meeting of our Patient Advisory Council. This medical practice advocate group has met regularly since 1974; it is made up of patients and health care professionals. Together they consult to provide health care services in a cost-effective manner, while preserving the personal nature of the doctor-patient relationship. They deal with issues of policy development, patient complaints, community education, patient-to-patient services, and practice management.

Our patients found the SF36 information to be a reasonably accurate reflection, but not particularly useful in and of itself, and offered numerous suggestions as to how it might be improved. This was somewhat surprising for an instrument whose psychometrics and quantitative methods are considered impeccable. In one eye-opening exchange, a patient said: "One thing I've learned about my own health is that spiritual health comes first, and I don't see any spiritual health component [here]."

Surely patients should have been more involved in the early design and testing of this instrument. Their collaborative participation might have been at least as important as the psychometric design.

THE PATIENT AS CORESEARCHER

In three other instances, we used our patients as research collaborators in the development of new applications.

In the first instance, we set out to develop a "language of negotiation" to describe comprehensive problem lists in a more efficient and collaborative way. As part of this effort, we wanted to eliminate terms that patients found difficult to define, difficult to understand, or demeaning. Over a period of several months, we asked patients to help us create terms to replace ones such as *neurotic, hypochondriac, schizophrenic,* and *psychopath*. Eventually, we were able to develop a language that was definable, less pejorative, less judgmental, and simpler (as judged by the Grade Equivalency Comprehension Scale). For example, to describe persons who resist treatment or advice, we eventually agreed on the term *patient role difficulty*. *Schizophrenia* became *reality disturbance; hypochondriasis* became *sensitive person and physical response to stress;* and *psychopath* became *impulse control deficiency and ethical violation of own standards*.

The second instance involved the development of a "spiritual health assessment" instrument. Here, we convened a focus group of patients who had each experienced a major personal calamity and asked them what their source of strength was. As we studied these personal narratives, we found words such as *acceptance, forgiveness, surrender,* and *willingness* and designed these into one section of our instrument. When we tested the instrument for internal consistency, this section showed the highest score, a result we attribute partially to the important contributions of our patient-collaborators. We also concluded that this form of collaboration in these two instances is necessary to understand some of the special issues such as communication and language.

In a third instance, we used focus groups to learn more about the effect on patients of our practice health educator. Here, we wished to solicit patients' opinions about this service and to compare their opinions with our own. We were working with the University of St. Thomas (in St. Paul, Minnesota) to develop a role definition, a curriculum, and a certification for this health educator, and we decided to consult with patients who had personally experienced this service.

The provider staff (physicians and health educators) identified patients with the following characteristics:

1. those perceived as difficult,
2. those who clearly had difficult problems, and
3. those who had experienced a successful outcome from the treatment process.

Out of 17 people identified, eventually 10 participated in the focus group. Patients were told that this was a discovery group, that its purpose was to discover how health care outcomes are achieved, and that we considered them colleagues in our search for how people get sick, and how they get well. A number of questions were posed that related to partnership, negotiation methods, reasons for good health behaviors, and the importance of family care, comprehensive care, and continuity of care.

The patients and their physicians occupied a circle of chairs, while three research observers sat outside of the circle and recorded their impressions with notes and tape recorders. Interaction between the observers and the focus group members was kept to a minimum. When the data collected by the observers were analyzed, patients seemed to be saying that, when their practitioners provided *listening and caring,* they in turn could provide *trust.* Trust led to *willingness,* and willingness led to better *participation* in the health care process. There was improved information exchange in the educational process, which in turn led to the *acquisition* of life management skills. It was these skills that *empowered* patients to take responsibility for and control of their own lives.

These patients talked about the importance to them of being treated in a holistic way, of receiving continuity of care over time, of being spoken to in a language that is understandable and as simple as possible, and of their practitioners focusing on their families as well as themselves. Although we didn't ask directly, three people in this group volunteered that they owed their lives to this collaborative, negotiatory style of health care delivery. Others may have had similar thoughts because this was a group of difficult people with difficult problems.

If the practitioner/patient relationship is important in health care services, it seems clear that it would take both parties working together to discover the deeper meanings and truths of this relationship. Did we do so in the case described above? We think so—in this instance, we learned in a practical way how practitioners can empower patients to follow a healing track. The assessment of interventions can be the same as the delivery of health care; or, said another way, ideally, research *is* health care. When doctors and patients are research collaborators within a practice setting, the research results can often be directly applied to the health care of those persons and to the care of subsequent patients as well.

QUALITY DESIGN FOR INTERVENTION ASSESSMENT RESEARCH

The primary care research professional has many tools, but practitioners, patients, and a community practice are among the most important. A quality design includes a clear understanding about organizing these resources, so that each component contributes its maximum value. At the base of this is shared language, negotiated consensus, and respectful collaboration.

Many research professionals are already taking these component parts seriously, but that is not enough. All three partners—the researcher, the practitioner, and the patient—must each take an active role, and this will not happen by accident. In practice, the researcher must actually *believe* in the power of this collaboration in order to seek out such involvement. It takes a minimum of belief to invite patients and practitioners into the data collection phase and a whole lot more to seek their participation in the phases of project design or data analysis.

As described, our group has had success with this approach, and we believe it holds rich potential. Perhaps it was easier for us because our Patient Advisory Council, which has participated in patient care and practice management since 1974, has created an atmosphere that includes valuing the participation of patients. It has been suggested that such a council or a community board is a key ingredient in the formation of a laboratory practice. (For discussions of these councils, see Cree, Lee, & Bates, 1982; Early, 1981; Early & Seifert, 1981; Naisbitt, 1982; Seifert, 1982, 1984, 1987.)

The clinical environment is the ideal laboratory in which to study family practice populations and develop new research methods. When such laboratories have ongoing collaborative relationships with universities, and when this interdependence becomes formally organized, then we will begin to see the full development of a primary care research methodology.

The motive behind this chapter has been that, based on our experience to date, we remain fearful that the potential of using qualitative designs and wide collaboration for assessing interventions will not graduate to reality.

References

Cree, J., Lee, L., & Bates, D. (1982). Negative physician response to patient participation in a family practice residency program. *Family Medicine, 14*, 4-7.

Early, F. D. (1981). Sharing practice management with patients. *Patient Care, 15*, 141-162.

Early, F., & Seifert, M. H. (1981). *Starting your own patient advisory council*. Spring Park, MN: M.D. Publishing.

Naisbitt, J. (1982). *Megatrends*. New York: Warner.

Seifert, M. H. (1982). The patient advisory council concept. In E. Connor & F. Mullan (Eds.), *Community oriented primary care* (Publication No. IOM-82-004). Washington, DC: National Academy Press.

Seifert, M. H. (1984). Patient advisory council cuts malpractice costs. *Patient Education Newsletter, 7*, 1-2.

Seifert, M. H. (1987). An incremental patient participation model. In P. A. Nutting (Ed.), *Community-oriented primary care: From principle to practice* (DHHS publication No. HRS-A-PE 86-1). Washington, DC: Government Printing Office.

Stewart, A. L., Hays, R. D., & Ware, J. E. (1988). The MOS short form general health survey: Reliability and validity in a patient population. *Medical Care, 26*(7), 724-735.

Wetzler, H. (1990). Recent applications of the SF-36. *CMS Update, 1*, 5.

10 Qualitative Designs
for Assessing Interventions
in Primary Care:
A Discussion

MARY-JO DELVECCHIO GOOD

Qualitative Research and Primary Care

In the past two decades, family medicine and primary care have matured as academic disciplines and have gained status as fields of specialization. The research traditions of internal and behavioral medicine that were incorporated into these new disciplines can thus now be examined through the lens of experience. Clinical epidemiology and experimental designs have dominated much of this research, with the drive for "p-values" and the fascination with quantitative data analysis shaping most research designs.

Yet researchers in these areas, having mastered the dominant quantitative models, are beginning to question the boundaries they establish (Miller & Crabtree, 1990; Stephenson, 1990). This questioning comes from a growing realization of the constraints and limits of these models and a concerted effort to explore other research paradigms. For example, physicians concerned with analyses of how experience is endowed with meaning—such as the meaning of symptoms to patients, the experience of illness for patients and their families, or the meaning and experience of clinical interactions for physicians—find qualitative methods of value.

The turn toward qualitative methodologies that is happening in family medicine in North America is concomitantly occurring among researchers in other disciplines and locales (see Coreil & Mull, 1981). Jerome Bruner (1986, 1990), one of the preeminent cognitive psychologists of our time, has turned to qualitative methodologies, in particular the analysis of narratives and stories, in his work on the psychology of thought. The Society of Behavioral Medicine devoted one of its keynote addresses in its March 1991 meeting to a critique of empiricist research models in medicine and to exploration of paradigms from interpretive medical anthropology (Geertz, 1973, 1983).

And, on the international health scene, young physician-researchers of Third World countries, who encounter brute facts of morbidity and mortality through their experiences in clinical and community medicine, find that many of their societies' health problems are resistant to assessment by traditional epidemiological methods and are turning instead to medical anthropology and qualitative methodologies.

Clinicians' Experience-Near Knowledge and Research

This questioning of traditional research methodologies appears to stem in part from the sense that clinical trials and epidemiology fail to tap into the complexities of medicine's clinical tasks and challenges. It also stems from a recognition that the kind of knowledge physicians gain from their daily clinical work, knowledge that we might label "experience-near knowledge" or "local knowledge," may be pragmatic and useful in shaping not only practice and interventions but research designs as well. (See Seifert, this volume.) The turn toward qualitative approaches suggests the emergence of new research paradigms, ones that take advantage of this type of knowledge and use it to formulate research questions and to structure research designs. The focus becomes a "bottom-up" rather than a "top-down" generation of research methodologies, with an emphasis on stories, texts, and meaning rather than on causal laws and hypotheses. That is, the definitions of problems and research designs become generated through everyday clinical practice and from the quandaries and questions that intrigue, engage, and sometimes baffle physicians.

As we evaluate what this turn toward qualitative methodologies means, we need to address the conceptual grounds that underpin research designs and methodological choices and to articulate what benefits such approaches could bring that are of consequence.

The examples presented by Janis Jenkins, Milton Seifert, and Dennis Willms address a number of these issues; indeed, their work suggests a somewhat revolutionary potential for crossing new research boundaries in primary care. Five issues emerge as critical to assessing the creative directions that qualitative approaches can bring:

1. the kinds of knowledge sought,
2. the fields of inquiry defined,
3. the methodological designs generated and used,
4. the modes of analysis and interpretation employed, and
5. the consequences both for clinical practice and for the design and assessment of interventions.

Toward a Meaning-Centered Approach to Research in Family Medicine

For more than a decade, a number of us who work at the interface of medicine and social science have proposed that medicine broaden its models to incorporate a "meaning-centered approach" to clinical practice (Eisenberg & Kleinman, 1981; Good & Good, 1981, 1982; Good, Good, Schaffer, & Lind, 1990; Kleinman, 1988; Kleinman, Eisenberg, & Good, 1977). This approach, which has relevance for research as well, assumes that the illness realities of patients are not simply defined by the somatic or psychophysiological dysfunctions from which they suffer. Rather, it emphasizes the importance of attaining *understanding* of these realities—of how patients and their families make sense of and attribute meaning to illness experiences and interactions with the medical profession. This knowledge requires attention to relevant data gained through qualitative methodologies, such as directive semistructured interviews, observations, and less formal discussions. The purposes of such methods are to elicit and evaluate patients' explanatory

Table 10.1 Comparison of the Biomedical and Cultural Hermeneutic
Models of Clinical Practice

Characteristics of the Biomedical (Empiricist) Clinical Model	Characteristics of the Cultural (Hermeneutic) Clinical Model
Pathological entity: Somatic or psychophysiological lesion or dysfunction	Meaningful construct, illness reality of the sufferer
Structure of relevance: Relevant data are those that reveal somatic disorder	Relevant data are those that reveal meaning of illness
Elicitation procedures: Review of systems, laboratory tests	Evaluate explanatory models, decode semantic network
Interpretive goal: Diagnosis and explanation	Understanding
Interpretive strategy: Dialectically explore relationship between symptoms and somatic disorder	Dialectically explore relationship between symptoms (text) and semantic network (context)
Therapeutic goal: Intervene in somatic disease process	Treat patient's experience: bring to understanding hidden aspects of illness reality and transform that reality

models of illness and to assess the process of development and the
dynamics of change in models; to listen to and analyze patients'
narratives and stories of illness; to attend to the affective and
interactional aspects of the illness experience and its changes over
course; and to decode the "semantic networks" of illness experience (see Table 10.1).

I define *semantic illness networks* as the concurrence of meanings
and experiences that are both individual and rooted in the larger
culture—such as the metaphors associated with a disease or symptoms, the popular lay theories about the illness, the culture's basic
values and concepts, and its forms of therapeutics, all of which
shape the experience of the illness and the social reactions to the

sufferer in a given family and society. These meanings emerge both in explanatory discourse and in narrative discourse—or through patients' stories.

In the clinical model, a central task includes an interpretive process, whereby the physician translates the patient's experiences into the context of the biomedical and clinical models of the medical profession. Intervention and therapeutics are aimed at teaching patients to confront their own networks of illness meanings and to assist them in the transformation of illness into health (or at least greater well-being).

While the meaning-centered approach has found its way into medical education and to some degree into clinical practice, its entry into medical research paradigms has been slower; research using this perspective has been largely conducted by medical anthropologists rather than by academics in family medicine or primary care. Recently, however, there has been considerable interest from researchers in these areas in applying this approach. (Postdoctoral fellows and visiting scholars at Harvard Medical School include primary care physicians who seek to broaden their research paradigms through studying medical anthropology.) An interest in narratives and in patients' stories has also fueled this focus on meaning and experience within the discipline (Brody, 1988; Kleinman, 1988; Miller & Crabtree, 1990). The study of smoking cessation reported by Dr. Willms (Chapter 8) is an excellent example of this in family medicine research, while Dr. Seifert (Chapter 9) not only describes qualitative methodologies of research in primary care practice but also suggests the importance of patient-generated designs and research agendas.

These new research paradigms in primary care do not pose too much of a design problem for those new to them—the elicitation of stories and the structuring of interviews are often quickly learned. But the analysis and interpretation of the qualitative data collected present a formidable challenge. Dr. Moira Stewart (in Willms et al., 1990) notes that qualitative data appear "less controlled."

In our own research with patients and physicians, we have analyzed the *culture* of medicine, using an interpretive approach that has flourished in the social sciences, particularly anthropology, for more than a decade. We have applied this perspective to the analysis of the meaning of symptoms to patients; to disclosure in

Table 10.2 A Cultural Model of Clinical Research

Elicit and evaluate patients' explanations, explanatory models of illness, and semantic networks of illness as related to experience of illness, action, and help seeking

Assess the dynamics of meanings of symptoms and illness/disease over time, including the development and change through the course of illness experience

Assess the physician's influence in shaping models of illness and therefore of experience of illness for patients through examining therapeutic narratives and affect/emotional tone in communication

Listen to and analyze patients' narratives, stories of illness experience

Attend to and record, through observation and interview, the affective and interactional aspects of illness experience and clinical encounters and the dynamics of change over course

American oncology and our culture's discourse on hope; to the meaning of physician competence in the practice of medicine, including conflicts between family medicine and obstetrics; and to therapeutic narratives—the way doctors shape the experience of illness course and treatment for patients through the stories and pacing that they construct in their clinical work and communications (see Table 10.2). I will return to therapeutic narratives shortly. (See Good & Good, 1981; Good et al., 1990; Mattingly, 1989.)

Knowledge, Inquiry, Analysis, Interpretation, and Consequences

In Chapters 7, 8, and 9, Drs. Jenkins, Willms, and Seifert reframe types of knowledge and fields of inquiry. Affect (emotional context), interactions, and meaning are central to their research designs.

Dr. Seifert (1987) focuses on how patients formulate what constitutes helpful action by their physicians, using the technique of focus group discussions, to bring out salient cultural models such as trust, listening, and willingness. His work is compelling in that it suggests future directions for research on physician-patient interactions, including the use of therapeutic narratives. It also raises a challenge as to how one interprets and analyzes findings from focus group discussions. What are appropriate levels of analysis? Dr. Seifert contrasts his group's findings and method with the limitations of quantitative assessment instruments designed outside community practice settings, and he drives home the significance of the emotional and affective dimensions of clinical work and of office-based research as well as the importance of affect in formulating research questions and designs.

Dr. Jenkins's (1991) research on expressed emotions as well as her chapter in this volume are suggestive of possible directions. Jenkins interviewed and observed relatives as they interacted with and discussed a mentally ill family member, then analyzed types of emotional expressions according to affective tone (for example, hostility, overinvolvement). Her finding was that illness course was significantly associated with and shaped by the affective tone of family interactions. This type of inquiry may identify areas for analysis of medical practice as well. Dr. Seifert's office-generated focus group study suggests that discussions among clinician-researchers and patients were laden with affect, which points to a potential area for future study of expressed emotion in clinical practice and care. A lesson may also be taken from Jenkins's work on expressed emotion in furthering assessment of the efficacy of various affective tones of physicians' therapeutic actions and narratives.

The work of Dr. Willms and his colleagues on the process of smoking cessation is a prime example of clinically relevant research that has its conceptual grounding in a meaning-centered research paradigm. In its focus on stories, it seeks to move beyond coded categorical data (a reassertion of control over data) to interpretations that tap into central dramas experienced by patients struggling to give up cigarettes. Rigor in this process stems from carefully crafted interview guidelines as well as from multiple levels of analysis, coding for themes, coding for affect, and analysis of the contiguity of meanings. Stories are analyzed for form, affect, dramatic content, and dilemmas as well as for key or recurring concepts. Willms's work also raises the very difficult issue of how analysis and interpretation should proceed and what qualitative methodologies imply about clinical practice and interventions. Table 10.3 summarizes processes of interpretation in a meaning-

Table 10.3 Meaning-Centered Analysis: The Interpretive Process

Decode semantic networks of illness experience and meaning
  (example: Willms this volume and Willms et al., 1990)

Analyze affect and expressed emotion in clinical encounters and between
patients and families
  (examples: Jenkins, Seifert, Willms—this volume)

Interpret modes of clinical interaction between physicians, patients, and families
  (examples: Jenkins, Seifert, Willms)

Categorize, analyze, and interpret types of illness stories of patients and correlate
with treatment experiences
  (example: Willms)

Analyze and assess physicians' therapeutic narratives over time and correlate
with patients' illness experience over course and outcome; correlate with outcome
  (see Seifert, who is beginning to address this)

Evaluate interventions in clinical care in terms of patient experience
  (examples: Seifert, Willms)

Formulate second stage of interventions
  (examples: Seifert, Willms)

centered analysis of clinical practice and clinical interactions and
interventions.

Therapeutic Narratives: An Additional Example

One field of inquiry that may attract the attention of family
medicine researchers is the narrative aspect of physician-patient
interactions. In the past decade, studies of patient-physician communication have used discourse analysis to identify power relationships between the voices of medicine and the patient's life
world as well as structures of relevance to the clinical context
(Mishler, 1984; Paget, 1982; Waitzkin, 1989; West, 1984; among
others). If we expand our research repertoires to include narrative
analysis, however, we would examine the stories not only of patients but also of physicians in the clinical encounter. We might
focus on how the latter use stories and narrative structures in the

process of treating patients and of shaping for them the experience and course of their disease. Dr. Seifert (this volume) makes a compelling argument for focusing on the beliefs and values of practicing clinicians, and analysis of physicians' therapeutic narratives may be one response to this challenge. For example, a study of oncologists (Good, 1990) noted that time horizons for patients are aggressively managed as part of the clinician's therapeutic task. Physicians deliberately blur or foreshorten time horizons to create experiences "for the moment" for cancer patients, especially those with serious prognoses. Similarly, Mattingly (1989) found that occupational therapists shape their patients' therapeutic experiences through the telling of stories about improvement of function; she refers to this activity as "therapeutic emplotment." Patients are told what to expect, are given tasks to pursue, are drawn into the drama of learning how to comb their hair again or to wheel themselves to the window. The therapist creates expectation and thereby shapes patient experience throughout the course of treatment.

If we similarly use the lens of narrative analysis to observe and analyze interactions between patients and their physicians, we can assess what types of therapeutic narratives are most efficacious. Types of narratives can be analyzed as to how they shape patients' experiences of healing or increasing wellness. In contrast to discourse or conversational analysis, which can often appear static, narrative analysis focuses on the process and dynamics of caring for patients over time (thus fitting with family medicine's philosophy of continuity of care). This emphasis on interaction between patient and physician makes sense both in the research world and in the clinical setting of primary care; such an approach does not focus solely on either party but seeks to capture the realities and veracities of everyday clinical work. The implications for research on interventions and in turn for medical training are potentially profound.

References

Brody, H. (1988). *Stories of sickness*. New Haven, CT: Yale University Press.
Bruner, J. (1986). *Actual minds, possible worlds*. Cambridge, MA: Harvard University Press.

Bruner, J. (1990). *Acts of meaning*. Cambridge, MA: Harvard University Press.

Coreil, J., & Mull, J. D. (Eds.). (1990). *Anthropology and primary health care*. Boulder, CO: Westview.

Eisenberg, L., & Kleinman, A. (Eds.). (1981). *The relevance of social science for medicine*. Dordrecht, Holland: D. Reidel.

Geertz, C. (1973). *The interpretation of cultures*. New York: Basic Books.

Geertz, C. (1983). *Local knowledge*. New York: Basic Books.

Good, B., & Good, M. (1981). The meaning of symptoms: A cultural hermeneutic model for clinical practice. In A. Kleinman & L. Eisenberg (Eds.), *The relevance of social science for medicine*. Dordrecht, Holland: D. Reidel.

Good, B., & Good, M. (1982). Toward a meaning-centred analysis of popular illness categories. In A. J. Marsellan & G. M. White (Eds.), *Cultural conceptions of mental health and therapy* (pp. 141-166). Dordrecht, Holland: D. Reidel.

Good, M. (1990, December). *Oncology and narrative time*. Paper presented at the American Anthropology Association Meeting, New Orleans, LA.

Good, M., Good, B., Schaffer, C., & Lind, S. (1990). American oncology and the discourse on hope. *Culture Medicine and Psychiatry, 14*, 59-79.

Jenkins J. (1991). Anthropology, expressed emotion and schizophrenia. *Ethos, 19*, 387-431.

Kleinman, A. (1988). *The illness narratives*. New York: Basic Books.

Kleinman, A., Eisenberg, L., & Good, B. (1977). Culture, illness and care. *Annals of Internal Medicine, 88*, 251-258.

Mattingly, C. (1989). *Thinking with stories: Stories and experience in a clinical practice*. Unpublished doctoral dissertation, Massachusetts Institute of Technology, Cambridge.

Miller, W. L., & Crabtree, B. F. (1990). Start with the stories. *Family Medicine Research Update, 9*, 2-3.

Mishler, E. (1984). *The discourse of medicine*. Norwood, NJ: Ablex.

Paget, M. (1982). Your son is cured now: You can take him home. *Culture, Medicine and Psychiatry, 6*(3), 237-259.

Seifert, M. H. (1987, May). *How do people get well?* Paper presented at the North American Primary Care Research Group Annual Meeting, Minneapolis, MN.

Stephenson, M. (1990). The relationship between family medicine and epidemiology. *Family Medicine Research Update, 9*, 1-2.

Waitzkin, H. (1989). A critical theory of medical discourse. *Journal of Health and Social Behavior, 30*, 220-239.

West, C. (1984). *Routine complications: Trouble with talk between doctors and patients*. Bloomington: Indiana University Press.

Willms, D. G., Best, J. A., Taylor, D. W., Gilbert, J. R., Wilson, D. M. C., Lindsay, E. A., & Singer, J. (1990). A systematic approach for using qualitative methods in primary prevention research. *Medical Anthropology Quarterly, 4*, 391-409.

PART III

Selected Topics
in Assessing Interventions
in Primary Care

Part III comprises much of the "main course" of the book, containing discussions of six prominent topics in primary care research interventions. Each topic is presented first with a discussion of its theory and then is followed by illustrative examples of original research.

The section begins with a chapter by Dr. Henry, an academic and educator on research skills for health professionals with extensive experience with self-report measures—a commonly used tool in primary care research. She offers a summary of survey technology, with many helpful pointers. Dr. Tudiver, a family physician and researcher, then describes two examples of his own use of self-report surveys, where one study used existing measures, and the other required the construction of new ones. The tasks involved and the pros and cons of each method are discussed.

Dr. Skinner, a professor of behavioral science, challenges readers to explore the issue of life-style assessment and change and its increasing prominence in primary care. He offers what he calls a "theoretical walkabout" of concepts of health and health care, detailing three issues in particular: how the determinants of health differ from those of disease; the difference between the notion of processes of changing health and the notion of processes of developing sickness; and appropriate levels of analysis (e.g., the individual versus the population).

Dr. Wilson, an academic family physician and researcher, describes his study of educational interventions with family physicians to change their clinical behavior with respect to aiding patients who smoke. His design is a useful example of how this sort of intervention with a common problem can be carried out and properly assessed.

Two analyses of assessing primary health care delivery follow. Dr. Williams, a researcher in clinical epidemiology, examines various studies of models of primary health care delivery, focusing on outcomes in terms of physician services, community health centers, and different payment schemes. Dr. Reid, a community-based family physician, reports on his study involving the analysis of interventions carried out by primary care physicians versus obstetricians in low-risk deliveries. Again, we have a good example of a feasible study of a common situation.

In the next chapter, Drs. Black, Roos (both researchers in population-based measurements of primary care), Rosser, and Dunn (both academic family physicians) focus on analyzing large data sets as a way to assess interventions. They describe two common sources—insurance company data and data sets developed in clinical practice—and they discuss the benefits and potential problems with each. Next, Dr. Dunn describes a study that analyzed an intervention in a rural setting (installation of a slow-scan video system to obtain long-distance diagnostic services) using a large data set of more than 150,000 encounters.

Drs. Oxman and Stachenko, both academic family practice researchers, present an overview of the theory and practice of performing meta-analyses on data from interventions and offer several examples that apply to primary care.

The last chapter in this section is by Dr. McWilliam, an academic nurse-researcher. She presents theoretical aspects of assessing primary care nursing interventions along with some examples and argues that, because much of what is important here has to do with the caring relationship between nurse and patient, new strategies need to be developed. The strategies discussed here are interpretive research, which uses various qualitative methodologies, and action research, which studies processes through changing them and observing the effect—a model already familiar to the nursing profession.

11 Self-Report Measures: Principles and Approaches

REBECCA HENRY

Self-report surveys are a popular research strategy in a diverse number of disciplines. For the researcher interested in understanding the complex areas of human thought and behavior, it would be difficult to imagine working without them.

There are generally three broad methods for collecting data:

Direct measurement involves quantification of the variable itself; for example, temperature can be measured with a thermometer; blood glucose with a glucometer.

Observation, where an external judge assesses overt behavior, can be conducted on a continuum, from highly structured and sociometric approaches to participant observation where the researcher is part of the event under investigation.

Interviewing, where the subject of study provides the required data through self-report, can occur in person, by telephone, or through the mail.

Virtually all these techniques have inherent strengths and weaknesses; none is free from error. This chapter summarizes specific characteristics of the *survey* as an instrument of measurement and discusses some principles for its use.

Definition and Characteristics of Surveys

While there is no universally accepted operational definition of a *survey*, Albreck and Settle (1985) identify many of its critical features as follows: "A survey is a research technique where informational requirements are specified, a population is identified, a sample selected and systematically questioned, and the results analyzed, generalized to the population and reported to meet the informational needs."

There is no better research technique when it comes to describing characteristics of human populations and understanding how they influence health, behavior, or cognition. Surveys may be used to collect information on a wide array of areas: knowledge, attitudes, behavior, demographic issues, health status, psychosocial conditions, symptoms, needs and demands, and affiliations.

Much research has been done on surveys themselves, drawing on the distinct methodological areas of sampling, instrumentation, data analysis and management, and report generation. The focus of this chapter is on the use of survey instruments and how they are often reported in the literature; the goal here is to understand what features one should look for in a survey instrument, and what are its strengths and weaknesses, especially for measuring the outcomes of intervention studies. For a comprehensive description of the steps required in the survey process, see Dillman (1978).

What Should You Look for in a Survey Instrument?

Whether you are in the process of developing a new instrument or assessing an existing one, there are a number of concerns you should have about its quality. Many investigators use surveys; however, too often these instruments were developed haphazardly, ignoring established standards. Two basic principles should always be adhered to: *theoretical grounding* and *empirical evaluation*.

THEORETICAL GROUNDING

In any research paradigm, there must be a meaningful linkage between theory, the research hypotheses, the research design, and instrument selection. When it comes to surveys, there should be an explicit relationship between the survey instrument and the theory that guides the research for which the survey is used. Unfortunately, too many investigators do not attend to this. Figure 11.1 describes the relationship between theory and methodology; this relationship serves as the foundation, guiding a particular research study as well as having an integrating function and linking different investigations. For example, in health promotion and disease prevention, one line of research examines the relationship of outcome expectations and self-efficacy to the likelihood of success in altering self-destructive behaviors; much of this research is a direct extension of Bandura's concepts of social learning theory in general and self-efficacy theory in particular (Bandura, 1977). Measures that are integrated with articulated theory make for more powerful research that can be aggregated into an organized framework and tested systematically. In arguing for the importance of a theoretical reference for instruments of self-report, Halvorsen (1990) asserts the following:

1. A theoretical framework provides the basis for construct definition, one important step in instrument development and evaluation.
2. Linking theory to instrument development causes investigators to be explicit about what they are measuring and how it is different than other constructs.
3. This approach allows for a more extensive evaluation of the scales developed for the instrument and for the constructs they represent.

EMPIRICAL EVALUATION

One cannot establish the appropriateness of a self-report instrument without evaluating its overall psychometric properties. This tells us how the instrument was constructed, and how it performed with a particular sample and under what conditions. In planning for the measurement of a specific outcome from an intervention, these qualities become critical. After all, if an instrument has low reliability and a high measurement error, it will not be sensitive to small or moderate changes on important dependent variables. Equally important, high variability of an instrument necessitates larger sample sizes to detect differences, thereby driving up the cost of the study.

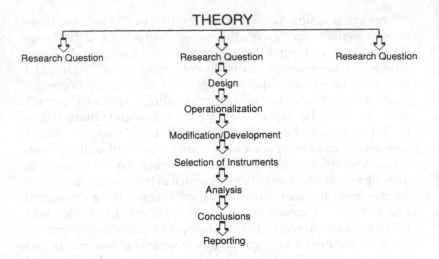

Figure 11.1. Relationship Between Theory and Methodology

The psychometric properties of the instrument often include the following:

- Item analysis
- Factor analysis
- Reliability assessment
    internal consistency
    alternate forms
    test retest
- Validity assessment
    concurrent
    predictive
    construct
- Norms
    scoring procedures
    population

For excellent overviews of the psychometric properties used in instrument development, the reader is referred to Volume 2 of the Research Methods for Primary Care series: Ferris and Norton (1992, "Basic Concepts in Reliability and Validity") and Zyzanski (1992, "Cutting and Pasting New Measures from Old"). Also, Nunnally

(1978) provides a comprehensive approach to the application of psychometric theory to instrument development.

Use of Surveys for Primary Care Research

As anyone who reads the research literature in primary care knows, surveys are a frequently used measure for dependent variables. There may be a number of reasons for this, some entirely appropriate and consistent with the research goal, others less so. Some of the advantages of using surveys for research in primary care are as follows:

- Surveys can be developed or customized to assess very specific outcomes of an intervention. (Because primary care is a relatively new and eclectic discipline, often a new measure must be created.)
- Most people are familiar with surveys and are able to complete them accurately.
- Surveys are often less expensive and less time-consuming than other methods for data collection.
- The self-reporting involved in surveys is the only way to collect many kinds of useful information (e.g., beliefs, needs, knowledge) that are at the heart of primary care research.

Disadvantages to using self-report surveys in primary care intervention studies exist too; however, rather than simply listing them, it may be helpful to present this topic in terms of some of the important issues researchers can expect to face.

(1) Should one use an existing measure or develop a new one? The chapters by Tudiver and Ferris (1992) and Zyzanski (1992) can help researchers determine which of these options is more appropriate. Whenever possible, it is always preferable to use an existing measure. First, new instruments are costly and time-consuming to develop; experts agree that one to two years' development time is not unusual. Second, developing a new instrument requires access to measurement experts, because rarely can a new investigator master psychometrics in addition to the competencies necessary to

implement an interventional study. Finally, generalizability among studies is difficult if researchers all select different instruments.

Unfortunately, often, existing instruments are not well suited to the specific purpose of an investigation or have never been used in a particular population or setting. If an instrument is incapable of detecting real change after treatment, it will be of no use at all. Therefore, on occasion, you *do* have to develop your own new instrument.

(2) What should the length be? The number of items to include in the instrument is an important question to consider. Unfortunately, the answer is never simple, as it incorporates both technical and nontechnical issues. There are, however, a few general guidelines to keep in mind:

- When developing and testing a new measure, begin with roughly twice the items you intend to have. Item analyses will help reduce the final number to a manageable set of questions.
- For unidimensional scales, good reliability often can be achieved with 20 to 30 items.
- Increasing the number of items increases the reliability of the instrument; however, there is a point of diminishing returns once reliability is moderate to high (.6-.8).
- In the planning stage, when conducting factor analyses, estimate that you will need roughly 6 to 10 subjects for every item tested. Experts don't always agree: Nunnally (1978) suggests 10:1; you may find others who consider a smaller number acceptable. In any event, it is not wise to use factor analysis with fewer than 100 subjects overall or fewer than 5 subjects per item as a planning guideline.
- The type of item format influences reliability. While it could take 30 dichotomous items to obtain a coefficient alpha of .80, one can often achieve that same level with 10 or so 7-point items on an agree/disagree scale.

The question of length is also influenced by other nontechnical factors. For example, do you want to measure one construct, or more than one? Fewer constructs can be measured more reliably. Too often, investigators elect to measure many different constructs, but none is measured particularly well.

Length can also influence response rates. If subjects perceive an instrument to be cumbersome or tiring, they often leave individual items unanswered or even fail to respond at all. Especially in the case of interventional studies in which subjects complete measures on multiple occasions, length needs to be carefully considered.

(3) Age-, sex-, and culturally appropriate measures. Because self-reports are often developed by academics who seem to communicate in their own dialect, items must be carefully examined for readability and population appropriateness. Frequently, we rely on our colleagues to edit and refine our items, and, unfortunately, they have the same biases we do. Recently, researchers have come to use focus groups in the early revision process. Employed frequently in the advertising profession, these groups consist of individuals representing the population of interest who discuss what the items mean to them and whether the words are meaningful and, if not, how they might be written more appropriately. If the focus group members are candid and comfortable in their roles, they can be an invaluable resource for developing new items. Another approach is to use readability indices to assess the level of difficulty of the words and sentences. These measures may be of some help although usually not as much as the direct feedback approach of focus groups.

(4) Content validity. Survey methodology and measures of self-report are used in a variety of different research designs: descriptive, correlational, and clinical trials. While in many ways the steps for instrument development or modification are fairly standardized, there is an important distinction to be made in the case of experiments or clinical trials where the essential goal is content validity (Nunnally, 1978, p. 312).

Investigators often confuse the different purposes of research designs. Many self-report measures are designed to describe features of particular groups or to correlate measures of one variable with measures of another—distinct purposes that require large, reliable individual differences on a particular attribute or construct but not at all necessary for measures to be used in clinical trials. For these, the issue should be one of developing a content-valid measure that is sensitive to the influence of the independent variable or intervention, that is, to differentiate treatment groups.

There is no quantitative measure for content validity; one always works toward improving it. Unlike other forms of validity, content validity is not correlated with a criterion or other measure, because the measure *is* the criterion. Content validity indicates whether the items in your instrument adequately sample a specific domain and whether they are constructed in the most appropriate form to test the content area. Content validity is therefore built into the measure development rather than assessed after it is completed. The process of ensuring content validity involves (a) obtaining a representative sample of items indicating the comprehensiveness of the construct, (b) involving experts in defining the construct and operationalizing critical terms, and (c) developing a format that is appropriate for the construct being assessed and a related scoring system.

Some work by Ware (1987) exemplifies these issues: In his efforts to develop valid measures for health, it became an essential focus to define what *health* actually is. Quality and quantity are certainly two dimensions, but what about others such as mental health and social functioning? Similarly, when devising rating scales, one must establish how to measure the responses and what the range of measurement should be. Ware states that many health scales emphasize a disease orientation, ignoring states of well-being. Measures that tap a comprehensive range of human responses are much more valid.

In summary, measures of self-report can be powerful tools for researchers investigating the complex domain of primary care. True, many surveys are poorly designed, lack empirical evaluation, or are not adequately documented; but, when done properly, surveys can be creative, psychometrically sound, and contribute substantially to what we know about health care and its delivery. If primary care researchers will make the effort to adhere to published standards for instrument development, now is an exciting time to participate in the generation of new knowledge and theory testing in this field.

References

Albreck, P., & Settle, R. (1985). *The survey research handbook*. Homewood, IL: Irwin.

Bandura, A. (1977). Self-efficacy: Toward a unifying theory of behavioral change. *Psychological Review, 84*, 191-215.

Dillman, D. (1978). *Mail and telephone surveys: The total design method*. Toronto: John Wiley.

Ferris, L. E., & Norton, P. G. (1992). Basic concepts in reliability and validity. In M. Stewart, F. Tudiver, M. J. Bass, E. V. Dunn, & P. G. Norton (Eds.), *Tools for primary care research.* Newbury Park, CA: Sage.

Halvorsen, J. (1990). Designing self-report instruments for family assessment. *Family Medicine, 22,* 478-484.

Nunnally, J. C. (1978). *Psychometric theory.* New York: McGraw-Hill.

Tudiver, F., & Ferris, L. E. (1992). Creating an original measure. In M. Stewart, F. Tudiver, M. J. Bass, E. V. Dunn, & P. G. Norton (Eds.), *Tools for primary care research.* Newbury Park, CA: Sage.

Ware, J. (1987). Standards for validating health measures: Definition and content. *Journal of Chronic Diseases, 40,* 473-480.

Zyzanski, S. J. (1992). Cutting and pasting new measures from old. In M. Stewart, F. Tudiver, M. J. Bass, E. V. Dunn, & P. G. Norton (Eds.), *Tools for primary care research.* Newbury Park, CA: Sage.

12 Using Instruments of Self-Report to Assess Interventions: Examples

FRED TUDIVER

In the previous chapter, Dr. Henry outlined some principles and approaches to consider when using self-report measures, especially surveys. This chapter presents two examples of the use of such measures in a primary care/community setting. The studies described here were concerned with mental health and behavior change topics, both relevant to the field of primary care. One study used existing measures; the other required the construction of new ones.

Example 1:
The "Widowers Surviving Project"

The objective of this community-based study was to assess the effectiveness of a mutual-help group intervention for new widowers (Tudiver, Hilditch, & Permaul, 1991; Tudiver, Hilditch, Permaul, & McKendree, 1992).

METHODS

Recent widowers in a large urban community were recruited to participate in a peer-group intervention focusing on health promotion. The men were randomly allocated to one of nine treatment groups or to a control group. The intervention consisted of nine weekly semistructured sessions that focused on issues such as the grief process, family, diet, new relationships, and physical exercise. Each group was led by two trained facilitators. Most of the facilitators in the study were themselves widowed and had experience in bereavement counseling. The design and analysis of this study, as well as those of the other study described, were carried out by primary care professionals. The sessions spent much of the time on sharing and venting feelings and on facilitating mutual support.

We wished to look at the effect of this intervention on psychological and social well-being by asking participants to complete self-administered measures. We used existing measures, for the following reasons: First, our group had limited resources and expertise with which to develop new ones, and, second, there were several existing instruments with theoretical grounding similar to our needs that had already been used to assess attributes of or interventions for the bereaved. The one significant drawback was that none had been used specifically to assess interventions for our population of interest (elderly widowers) to any great extent.

The following self-report instruments were selected: (a) The 28-item Goldberg General Health Questionnaire (Goldberg, 1978) rates psychoemotional distress in terms of everyday functioning. It had previously been used to evaluate the benefits of mutual-help interventions for widows (Vachon, Lyall, Rogers, Greedman-Letofsky, & Freeman, 1980) but not for widowers. (b) The 13-item short form of the Beck Depression Inventory (Beck & Beck, 1972; Beck, Ward, Mendelson, Mock, & Erbaugh, 1961) measure of depression has been used in primary care settings and for evaluating the benefits of mutual help for widows (Marmar, Howowitz, Weiss, Wilner, & Kaltreider, 1988). (c) The 42-item Social Adjustment Scale (Weissman & Bothwess, 1976; Weissman, Prusoff, Thompson, Harding, & Myers, 1978) is designed to evaluate treatment for psychotherapy by assessing social areas such as work outside and in the home, spare time, family, and children. It has been used for evaluating the benefits of mutual help for widows (Marmar et al., 1988). (d) The 27-item Social Support Questionnaire (Sarason, Levine, Basham, & Sarason, 1983) is designed to quantify the availability of, and satisfaction with, social support. (e) The 20-item State-Anxiety Inventory (STAI; Spielberger, 1983) asks how respondents are feeling at that particular moment.

All the measures were administered at baseline (before random-ization), at the end of the 9-week intervention period, and 6 months postintervention (8 months postrecruitment). Subjects reported a few problems with the measures. The most common complaints were that they took too long to complete (at least one hour) and that the instructions were difficult to follow, in particular those for multiple-choice responses. (Many of these elderly men had had little or no prior experience with this type of measure.) In addition, many complained that items and even entire scales were not rele-vant to their situation and that they disliked "completing different questionnaires that kept asking me the same questions" (e.g., the Beck Depression Inventory and the General Health Questionnaire).

RESULTS

There were no significant differences between treatment subjects and controls at baseline. Group-by-time ANOVAS over the three observations showed no improvements due to the intervention; in fact, the trend was in the opposite direction, with all psychological scores for the control subjects showing greater improvement over time. The scores on the STAI were statistically significantly higher (a higher score means more anxiety) over the time period in the treatment groups.

Example 2:
"The Talking Sex Project"

In this community-based study, we conducted a randomized controlled trial of an AIDS risk reduction program for gay and bisexual men (Myers et al., 1992; Tudiver et al., 1992).

METHODS

Gay and bisexual men from a large urban community were invited to participate in a peer-group health education interven-tion. We had to marshal all our creativity to recruit our subjects; venues included gay bars, baths, and social events; advertisements and media reports; word of mouth; posters, pamphlets, buttons, and mailings sent to community groups, clinics, and physicians; and physician referrals.

The subjects, who practiced sexual behavior at all ranges of risk for transmission of HIV, were randomly assigned to one of two treatment interventions or to a waiting-list control group. The interventions comprised either one 2-hour peer-group evening meeting (single session) facilitated by two trained peers (gay men) or four weekly 1.5-hour peer-group meetings (serial session) facilitated by two trained professionals, mostly nonpeer (a man and a woman) leaders. Much of the group time was spent on education about AIDS prevention and on communicating and sharing experiences and feelings on this topic.

To measure the effect of the interventions on knowledge, attitudes, and sexual practices with respect to AIDS prevention, we administered questionnaires both at baseline (before randomization) and 3 months after the completion of the interventions. Several self-report measures on these issues already existed, but few had known psychometric properties or had been used to assess an educational intervention in this area. We therefore created and tested our own instrument, partly by cutting and pasting items from these existing ones. This undertaking took a great deal of effort, and almost 2 years' work, but a major benefit was our confidence that we had a measure with known psychometric properties for our particular population.

RESULTS

There was a significant improvement in knowledge of AIDS risk over time for all groups, with the two treatment groups showing the largest gains (analyzed by 3×2 group $\times$ time repeated measures ANOVA for group comparison; $F = 4.80$, df = 2,472, $p < .0087$). With respect to attitudes about AIDS prevention, our greatest interest was in items relating to a construct we named "Condom Efficacy," based on Bandura's (1987) concept of "self-efficacy" (Bandura, 1987): an individual's belief in his or her own capability to change health-care-related behavior. There was a significant improvement in the mean scores for Condom Efficacy items for all groups, with the two treatment groups showing the greatest improvement ($F = 3.06$, df = 2,479, $p < .048$).

The results of the study's primary outcome—change to practice of safer sex—were not as clear. Of those who changed their sexual practices, there was an overall trend toward safer sex. This shift was strongest in the single-session group, but there was no statistically significant group-by-time interaction for this outcome. We were not able to come up with an explanation for this result.

Discussion

Each of these two studies used self-administered measures as the most satisfactory, acceptable, and affordable method for collecting sensitive and confidential data.

In the AIDS study, the construction of a new measure had several advantages. The most important of these was the assurance of excellent content and face validity, because the instrument was devised to address particular research questions and was pretested on a sample of the targeted population.

Creation of the original measure, however, which required much time, energy, and money to construct, test, and refine, was only possible because of generous federal government resources. This sort of undertaking is often beyond the scope and available resources of primary care researchers.

The "Widowers Surviving Project" suffered from the fact that many of the measures used in it had been developed and validated on diverse populations, several of which did not resemble our study population. The instruments were burdened with unrelated or inappropriate items, and sometimes different measures asked the same questions. In two poststudy focus groups, we discovered that a number of dropouts had occurred because of resistance to these two frequently complained about problems. In addition, many of the men complained about having to complete the same measures on four different occasions.

An important issue for both studies is whether the measures used in them were sensitive enough to detect the differences we were seeking. In the focus group sessions that followed the intervention with widowers, men in the treatment groups were assessed by four independent raters as being less depressed and anxious than their control group counterparts; however, the quantitative measures indicated the opposite trend (although not to a significant degree).

In the AIDS study, analyses of data showed beneficial treatment effects on knowledge and on some attitudes but difficult-to-explain effects—and noneffects—on behavior. The investigators concluded that variables such as group leadership may have provided important biases here but that the self-administered measures were probably not sensitive to these issues. It is possible that a face-to-face interview-type measure or several focus groups may have revealed more information.

The participants in the focus groups of the widowers project revealed that the rather high dropout rate of the widowers was in part due to the *nature* of instrument administration. About half the measures were administered face-to-face during the orientation and final treatment sessions, but the rest had to be mailed. (In the AIDS project, all subjects had their measures administered face-to-face, which may partly account for their relatively high participation rate of 82%; however, it is difficult to make comparisons between two different studies involving two very different populations.) There are pros and cons to both approaches: Administering a self-report measure face-to-face often creates more anxiety, especially in a group setting, whereas one that is mailed can be completed in the subject's own private space and time; however, it is more difficult to achieve high return rates with mailed surveys. In addition, mailing presents its own peculiar difficulties. For example, using registered mail instead of regular delivery often results in higher and quicker return rates, but the costs are several times higher. In addition, the timing of the successive steps in a mailed system of administration is important: It is crucial to determine the turnaround times of your catchment area's mail delivery to plan an optimal schedule for your mailings. (For a discussion of other important factors that are beyond the scope of this chapter to consider, see, for example, Dillman, 1978; Sudman & Bradburn, 1983; Tudiver & Ferris, 1992.)

Summary

Self-report measures are one of the most commonly used instruments in primary care research. The two examples in this chapter illustrate how such measures can be used by primary care researchers to assess interventions and also indicate several of their important advantages, disadvantages, and problems. The major advantages are that they are efficient and useful for collecting sensitive and personal data: Those that already exist are available and economical, and those that are created for a particular intervention study are likely to ensure good content and face validity.

An important disadvantage is they can be insensitive to the treatment effect being sought. This is a particular problem with existing measures that were created for different populations; however, attempts to minimize this problem and improve construct validity by creating an original measure can be expensive and time-consuming. Another problem experienced in the example studies was the effect of instrument administration on the dropout rate, specifically the effects of mailed instruments and repeated administrations.

In sum, while the use of self-administered measures to assess an intervention can be of great value, their sole use may yield insufficient data to explain the results. This may be an important matter to consider, especially in primary care intervention studies of behavior change or mental health issues. Studies in this area will often require the added thickness or enhancement of the data beyond that which is provided by limited paper-and-pencil instruments of self-report. We therefore recommend that researchers use qualitative measures like face-to-face interviews as well as focus groups to supplement their data derived from self-report.

References

Bandura, A. (1987). Self-efficacy: Toward a unifying theory of behavioral change. *Psychological Review, 84*, 191-215.

Beck, A. T., & Beck, R. W. (1972). Screening depressed patients in family practice: A rapid technic. *Postgraduate Medicine, 52*, 81-85.

Beck, A. T., Ward, C. H., Mendelson, M. M., Mock, J., & Erbaugh, J. (1961). An inventory for measuring depression. *Archives of General Psychiatry, 4*, 561-571.

Dillman, D. A. (1978). *Mail and telephone surveys: The total design method*. Toronto: John Wiley.

Goldberg, D. (1978). *Manual of the General Health Questionnaire*. Windsor, England: NFER.

Marmar, C. R., Howowitz, M. J., Weiss, D. S., Wilner, N. R., & Kaltreider, N. B. (1988). A controlled trial of brief psychotherapy and mutual-help group treatment of conjugal bereavement. *American Journal of Psychiatry, 145,* 203-209.

Myers, T., Tudiver, F., Kurtz, R. G., Orr, K., Rowe, C., Jackson, E., & Bullock, S. L. (1992). The Talking Sex Project: Descriptions of the study population and correlates of unsafe sexual practices at baseline. *Canadian Journal of Public Health, 83*(1), 47-52.

Sarason, I. G., Levine, H. M., Basham, R. B., & Sarason, B. R. (1983). Assessing social support: The Social Support Questionnaire. *Journal of Personality and Social Psychology, 44,* 127-139.

Spielberger, C. D. (1983). *Manual for the State-Trait Anxiety Inventory.* Palo Alto, CA: Consulting Psychologists Press.

Sudman, S., & Bradburn, N. M. (1983). *Asking questions: A practical guide to questionnaire design.* San Francisco: Jossey-Bass.

Tudiver, F., & Ferris, L. (1992). Creating a new measure. In M. Stewart, F. Tudiver, M. Bass, E. V. Dunn, & P. Norton (Eds.), *Tools for primary care research.* Newbury Park, CA: Sage.

Tudiver, F., Hilditch, J., & Permaul, J. (1991). A comparison of psychosocial characteristics of new widowers and married men. *Family Medicine, 23,* 501-505.

Tudiver, F., Hilditch, J., Permaul, J., & McKendree, D. J. (1992). Does mutual-help facilitate newly bereaved widowers? Report of a randomized controlled trial. *Evaluation & the Health Professions, 15*(2), 147-162.

Tudiver, F., Myers, T., Kurtz, R. G., Orr, K., Rowe, C., Jackson, E., & Bullock, S. (1992). The Talking Sex Project: Results of a randomized controlled trial of small group AIDS education for 612 gay and bisexual men. *Evaluation & the Health Professions, 15*(4), 26-42.

Vachon, M. L. S., Lyall, W. A., Rogers, J., Greedman-Letofsky, K., & Freeman, S. J. (1980). A controlled study of self-help intervention for widows. *American Journal of Psychiatry, 137,* 1380-1384.

Weissman, M. M., & Bothwess, S. (1976). Assessment of social adjustment by patient self-report. *Archives of General Psychiatry, 33,* 1111-1115.

Weissman, M. M., Prusoff, B. A., Thompson, W. D., Harding, P. S., & Myers, J. K. (1978). Social adjustment by self-report in a community sample and in psychiatric outpatients. *Journal of Nervous and Mental Diseases, 166,* 317-326.

13 Life-Style Assessment and Change: Theory, What Theory?

HARVEY A. SKINNER

Life-style issues have captivated public attention. A perusal of any bookstore or television talk show will reveal the latest strategies for losing weight, keeping fit, eating better, avoiding stress, quitting smoking, drinking less, and enjoying life more! Some popular self-help books include *The Joy of Stress* (Hanson, 1985), *The Well Audit* (Samuels & Samuels, 1988), and *A Wellness Way of Life* (Robbins, Powers, & Burgess, 1991).

In the past two decades, life-style assessment and change have assumed increasing importance in primary care. Patients expect their doctor to assess and be knowledgeable about their life-style habits and to provide appropriate assistance and counseling when necessary (Schwenk, Clark, Jones, Simmons, & Coleman, 1982; Wallace & Haines, 1984). There has been a proliferation of techniques for conducting life-style assessments, such as the health hazard appraisal and health risk approaches (DeFriese & Fielding, 1990; Weiss, 1984). From the physician's perspective, surveys have found that most physicians believe it is very important to educate their patients about life-style behaviors, such as smoking, diet and weight control, alcohol use, and exercise (Sobal, Valente, Muncie, Levine, & Deforge, 1985). Yet, many physicians do not routinely gather such information (Wallace & Haines, 1984; Wechsler, Levine, Idelson, Rohman, & Taylor, 1983).

Despite the oftentimes missionary zeal surrounding life-style assessment and change, it is highly instructive to take a step back and consider the underlying assumptions. This chapter presents an overview of conceptual issues: a "theoretical walkabout." Changing concepts of health and health care are reviewed. A particular focus is on the increasing recognition that the determinants of health (*salutogenesis*) are often different than the determinants of disease (*pathogenesis*). Another important distinction explored here is how different concepts are generally needed for understanding how to *change* a health condition (processes of change) than are needed for understanding how the condition *developed*. A third focus is on the appropriate level of analysis, such as individual versus population perspectives on health.

Theory, What Theory?

From the outset, one must recognize that most health behavior research proceeds without a strong theoretical grounding. We are a long way from having "scientific" theories in which the constructs have clearly specified theoretical linkages and unambiguous empirical definition or measurement (Meehl, 1978). Most "theories" in this area are not couched in a form that is readily open to empirical evaluation and falsification (Phillips, 1987) and should be viewed either as conceptual models (lacking strong theoretical specification and empirical definitions) or even as mere heuristics. Much of the research would appear to be atheoretical (e.g., surveys), where no conceptual framework is evident as a guide for the selection of questions and interpretation of results. The situation is even worse in the sense that the predominant approach to science in the Western hemisphere (quantitative, positivism) is being seriously challenged (Baldus, 1990; Bryman, 1984).

One might conclude the chapter at this point and simply state: Theory, what theory? On the other hand, this discussion is fruitful if the reader is sensitized to the relatively early or immature state of theory and research regarding health behavior. Also, there are some very exciting developments with respect to evolving concepts of health and models for change at both the individual and the population levels. Herein lie the seeds of concepts that may one day blossom into scientific theories.

Evolving Concepts of Health Promotion

There is an old maxim, well understood by politicians, that how an issue gets *defined* influences our *understanding* of it, which in turn influences our *behavior*. This maxim is particularly relevant to health care, where a remarkable shift in emphasis is beginning to occur. The traditional, almost exclusive focus on curative medicine and high technology is being seriously challenged (Roemer, 1984). Concepts of health and health care are being redefined, which is setting the stage for broad changes in our understanding and behavior.

The 1970s ushered in the era of focusing on individual life-style choices. An international milestone was the publication in Canada of the Lalonde report (1974), which differentiated among four interlinked determinants of health: human biology, life-style, environment, and the health care system. These concepts had a major impact upon the U.S. Surgeon General's report in 1979 titled *Healthy People* and on the subsequent *Promoting Health, Preventing Disease: Objectives for the Nation* (U.S. Department of Health & Human Resources, 1980). When experts analyzed the 10 leading causes of death in the United States, their findings underscored the importance of life-style: Approximately 50% of mortality in 1976 was due to unhealthy behavior or life-style, 20% to environmental factors, 20% to human biological factors, and 10% to inadequacies in health care (U.S. Surgeon General, 1979). The tenor of the time is perhaps best captured in the following quotation from J. A. Califano in the report: "We are killing ourselves by our own careless habits. You, the individual, can do more for your own health and well-being than any doctor, any hospital, any drug, any exotic medical device" (U.S. Surgeon General, 1979).

This emphasis on life-styles led to the development of assessment procedures such as health hazard appraisal and to interventions such as physicians' advice to patients about cigarette smoking (e.g., Russell, Wilson, Taylor, & Baker, 1979). Prospective studies, such as the 9-year Alameda County project (Berkman & Breslow, 1983), showed that simple life-style habits can significantly reduce the risk of disease and mortality, such as not smoking cigarettes, moderate or no alcohol use, maintaining desirable weight, regular physical exercise, 7-8 hours sleep each night. Nevertheless, many critics (e.g., Levin, 1987) argued that the emphasis on individual life-style change was being oversold ("blaming the victim"). Consequently, a rebalancing of focus to population and structural determinants of health occurred in the 1980s.

At the international level, in its Declaration of Alma Ata, the World Health Organization (1978) proposed a wider concept of health as being not merely an end in itself but a resource for living. This declaration was followed by the commitment to "Health for All," where emphasis was placed on primary and community-based health care, appropriate technology, community involvement, and multisectoral approaches. At the first international conference on health promotion held in Ottawa, Canada, in 1986, a Charter for Action was adopted for the achievement of health for all by the year 2000 and beyond (WHO, 1986). The Ottawa charter emphasizes five interdependent actions:

1. Build healthy public policy
2. Create supportive environments
3. Strengthen community action
4. Develop personal skills
5. Reorient health services

As we move into the 1990s, there is still an appreciation of the importance of clinical prevention initiatives, but there has been an important corrective factor for the overemphasis on individual change that was promulgated in the 1970s. Life-style assessment and change is just one strategy, among many, of a comprehensive approach to health and health care that includes community action and environmental and public policy domains. In Canada, these broader concepts are incorporated into a national framework for health promotion titled "Achieving Health for All" (Epp, 1986).

Focus of Theory

Researchers and clinicians in primary care must look with some bewilderment at the diverse array of theory and models about health behavior. No single perspective has gained ascendance, and there is a pressing need for a general framework that would provide coherence for this field. One helpful step in this direction is the analytic framework recently proposed by Evans and Stoddart

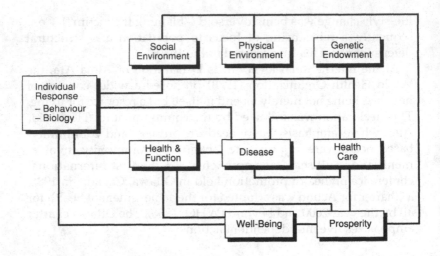

Figure 13.1. Framework for Understanding Health
SOURCE: Reprinted with permission from Evans & Stoddart, 1990, Pergamon Press, Ltd.

(1990). Their analysis begins with a simple framework involving disease and health care; the framework is then built up, component by component, by addressing inadequacies of the preceding stage. The final model (see Figure 13.1) includes individual responses (e.g., life-style), the social and physical environments, and structural considerations such as prosperity, individual functional capacity, and concepts of health and well-being. This analysis provides an excellent "road map" of the comprehensive factors involved in health behavior.

The following section considers three aspects that are particularly relevant to primary care.

DETERMINANTS OF HEALTH VERSUS ILLNESS

Traditionally, most of the theory and interest in "health" has actually been directed at understanding the determinants of illness, disease, and disability. A basic assumption of this pathogenic paradigm is homeostasis, which may be disrupted by biological and/ or psychosocial factors (Antonovsky, 1984). To restore homeostasis, regulatory mechanisms such as the neurological, immune, and endocrine systems come into play. When these mechanisms are inadequate, disease results and medical intervention is sought to restore homeostasis. Reconceptualizations of the traditional medical model, such as Engels's (1977) biopsychosocial model, are still predominantly focused on understanding the determinants of illness.

An alternative perspective is to focus on understanding the determinants of *good* health, or "salutogenesis" (Antonovsky, 1979). Why do so many individuals remain healthy, even in the presence of disease-producing pathogens in their bodies and environments? Different factors may propel an individual toward one end (pathology) or the other (health) of the continuum. A focus on understanding the determinants of health is embodied in the World Health Organization definition of health as "a state of complete physical, mental, and social well-being—not merely the absence of disease or infirmity" (WHO, 1978). An important consequence of this new definition is recognition of the importance of the social, political, and economic environments. With this new approach, health now encompasses work in areas such as income and economic disparity, peace, education, and the cultural environment.

UNDERSTANDING VERSUS CHANGING
HEALTH BEHAVIOR

There are a variety of models that attempt to explain health behavior. One, the Health Belief Model (Becker, 1974), has attracted considerable attention. This model proposes that the likelihood of an individual undertaking any health behavior is a function of (a) the perceived magnitude of a threat to his or her health (belief in personal susceptibility, anticipated severity of the disease) and (b) the perception of the relative efficacy of a specific behavior in dealing with that threat. This model has been criticized for its lack of conceptual rigor and its relatively poor predictive power (Norman, 1986).

An alternative model is the Theory of Reasoned Action (Fishbein & Ajzen, 1975), which proposes that a sufficient predictor of voluntary action is immediate behavioral intention and that such intentions are a function of (a) attitude toward the act and (b) subjectively perceived norms concerning the act. That is, the more

STAGES

LEVELS   1. Precontemplation   3. Action
                        2. Contemplation   4. Maintenance

a) Symptoms

b) Cognitions   PROCESSES OF CHANGE

c) Interpersonal   e.g., • Helping relationship
                                  • Consciousness-raising
d) Family/Systems   • Stimulus control

e) Intrapersonal

Figure 13.2. Comprehensive Model of Change
SOURCE: Adapted from Prochaska and DiClemente (1986).

that an individual evaluates an act positively and/or believes that significant others favor it, the greater the likelihood that he or she will perform it. With respect to health behavior, empirical evidence suggests that the Theory of Reasoned Action is capable of predicting more variance than the Health Belief Model (Norman, 1986).

A third model that has attracted considerable interest and support is Self-Efficacy Theory (Bandura, 1977; Schunk & Carbonari, 1984). Its key element is that self-referent thoughts mediate the relationship between knowledge and action; that is, people self-regulate their environments and actions. Bandura has proposed that the central element of self-referent thinking is an individual's perception of his or her *self-efficacy*; that is, the sense of "I can do."

In contrast, other models focus primarily on understanding the processes of change. An example here is the Comprehensive Model of Change proposed by Prochaska and DiClemente (1986), which emphasizes three components of change: stages, processes, and levels (see Figure 13.2). In a comparison of persons who were either self-changers or participated in a treatment program (therapy change), four common *stages of change* were identified: precontemplation, contemplation, action, and maintenance. Most people do not progress in a linear fashion through these stages of change; instead, relapses are common and one may recycle from relapse (maintenance) back through contemplation and action stages. "Precontemplators" may be largely unaware that a particular behavior (e.g., a fast-food, high fat diet) may have long-term implications for their health (e.g., heart disease). The chronic "contemplator" may for many years talk about changing a life-style behavior (e.g., losing weight, quitting smoking, starting an exercise program, cutting down on drinking) but does not take concrete action to initiate this change. With respect to cigarette smoking, self-changers make at least three serious revolutions through the stages of change before they achieve long-term abstinence. A basic hypothesis is that change is most likely to occur if both the client (patient) and the therapist (physician) are focusing on the same stage of change.

In examining what individuals do to progress from one stage to the next, Prochaska and DiClemente proposed 10 basic *processes of change*. The three most frequently used processes across a variety of problem areas included (a) helping relationships, (b) consciousness-raising, and (c) self-liberation. Some interesting interactions were noted. For example, helping relationships and consciousness-raising were more frequently used for dealing with psychological distress, while weight-control subjects tended to rely more on self-liberation and stimulus control techniques. Another important finding was that different processes are relevant at different stages of change. Consciousness-raising is most relevant when moving from contemplation to action. During the action stage, self-liberation is important for underscoring the individual's sense that his or her own efforts play a critical role in successful behavioral change (sense of self-efficacy). Preparation for the maintenance phase is enhanced by counterconditioning and stimulus control processes.

The third component of this model involves levels of *change*. Prochaska and DiClemente propose a hierarchical organization of five distinct but interrelated levels (Figure 13.2), and it is important that the therapist and client are focusing upon the same level or levels. Usually, an individual seeks help because of a particular problem (symptom/situational level). Different schools of therapy have different theoretical perspectives on what level of change is most appropriate. For instance, behaviorists tend to focus on the symptom and situational determinants; family therapists focus on the family system's level; and psychoanalytic therapists focus on intrapersonal conflicts. Because of the time pressure in primary care settings, attention generally focuses at the symptom/

situational level. Referral for specialized help is generally required as one moves deeper down the level that needs to be changed.

WHAT IS THE APPROPRIATE LEVEL OF ANALYSIS?

In his monumental book *Living Systems*, Miller (1978) uses general systems theory to show how biological and social systems are organized and operate at seven hierarchical levels:

1. Cells
2. Organs (composed of cells)
3. Organisms (independent life forms)
4. Groups (families, committees)
5. Organizations (communities, cities, corporations)
6. Societies (nations)
7. Supranational systems (e.g., the European Common Market)

Miller postulated 19 subsystems at each level that are essential for life, some of which process matter or energy, and some information. The complexity of the system increases as one advances deeper into the hierarchy from the cellular level.

Most of us tend to focus our work within a given level, although we may at times make journeys one level up or one level down the hierarchy. This tends to be the limit of our theoretical "comfort zone." For example, I am a psychologist by training, and the brunt of my research has been concerned with the individual (organism). For example, I have focused on the development of instruments for the early identification and assessment of alcohol/drug problems. At certain points in my career, I have traveled one level down the hierarchy, where I have studied various organ systems, particularly the liver. My interest is in whether certain liver enzymes (e.g., GGT) may be useful as laboratory markers of alcohol use by an individual (Skinner, Holt, Sheu, & Israel, 1986). This research would not have been possible without the collaboration of a biochemist (Israel) and a gastroenterologist (Holt). I have also ventured in the other direction, however, one step up the hierarchy, to the level of the family group. Here, I have worked with colleagues from psychiatry and social work in attempting to understand how family interactions may precipitate, maintain (enable), or be influenced by the health behavior of a given family member (Skinner, 1987; Steinhauer, Santa-Barbara, & Skinner, 1984).

Conceptual developments with respect to health promotion certainly present us with immense challenges in dealing with different levels of analysis. For instance, the Ottawa charter forces one to examine various levels running from the individual (e.g., personal skills) through to the family, the community, the health care system, the physical and social environment, and public policy, which cuts across all levels. The important points are to appreciate the spectrum of levels, to be specific about what particular level or levels one is addressing, and to avoid professional snobbery and intolerance of those who work at a different level in the hierarchy.

In primary care, one is often faced with the question of whether health behavior interventions should focus on the individual or the population (community) level. A key to resolving this issue is to understand the *prevention paradox* (Rose, 1981). That is, an intervention that helps a relatively small number of "at-risk" individuals (e.g., physician advice against smoking) is unlikely to offer great benefits to the population. Conversely, a measure that offers substantial benefits to the population (e.g., seat-belt legislation) is less likely to have immediate impact on individual behavior (seat-belt use rates in Canada have increased from 36.4% in 1980 to 75.8% in 1988; Transport Canada, 1990). Neither approach is optimal.

Jeffery (1989) reviews the conditions under which individual strategies are most effective: (a) benefits to the individual are large; (b) time interval when the individual will benefit is short; and (c) effort to change the behavior is low, relative to the expected benefit. Notable successes include the adoption of birth control devices to prevent unwanted pregnancies and the use of fluoridated toothpaste to prevent dental caries. In comparison, population (community) approaches to health behavior change are most effective when (a) the environmental context is well defined where the behavior occurs, (b) the health behavior is in the public domain, and (c) intervention is politically and economically feasible. Illustrations of successful population approaches include environmental engineering (e.g., water sanitation) and safety regulation (e.g., building codes, regulation of prescription drugs). In most cases, individual and population strategies are mutually supportive and can be used together to create a public climate of expectancy about health risk behaviors. For instance, the decline in cigarette smoking in the past two decades has resulted from a complex interplay of individual and population factors.

Conclusion

I will conclude with a caution that is voiced by colleagues in sociology and philosophy, who remind us of pitfalls in the logic of scientific research. Contextual factors can influence our essential definitions and concepts—our worldview (Phillips, 1987). This point is amply illustrated by a recent "experiment" with my 7-year old daughter, Ana, who is at the age when children lose their baby teeth. Ana was away the previous night for a sleep-over at a friend's house when one of her front teeth came out. The next morning, she returned home in a great state of distress. The Tooth Fairy had forgotten to leave money under her pillow in exchange for her tooth. Oh dear! That night I diligently helped Ana craft this letter (an intervention?): "Dear Tooth Fairy: If you don't leave me anything I won't believe in you. From Ana."

The next morning, Ana came rushing into my bedroom with a big gap-toothed smile on her face and a $1 bill in her hand. "Daddy, look what the Tooth Fairy brought me." I also smiled as I lay back in bed and pondered how this evidence supported our theories about the existence of the Tooth Fairy.

References

Antonovsky, A. (1979). *Health, stress and coping*. San Francisco: Jossey-Bass.
Antonovsky, A. (1984). The sense of coherence as a determinant of health. In J. D. Matarazzo, S. M. Weiss, J. A. Herd, N. E. Miller, & S. M. Weiss (Eds.), *Behavioral health: A handbook of health enhancement and disease-prevention* (pp. 114-129). New York: John Wiley.
Baldus, B. (1990). Positivism's twilight? *Canadian Journal of Sociology, 15,* 149-163.
Bandura, A. (1977). Self-efficacy: Toward a unifying theory of behavioral change. *Psychological Review, 84,* 191-215.
Becker, M. H. (1974). The Health Belief Model and personal health behavior. *Health Education Monographs, 2,* 326-473.
Berkman, L. F., & Breslow, L. (1983). *Health and ways of living: The Alameda County Study*. New York: Oxford University Press.
Bryman, A. (1984). The debate about quantitative and qualitative research: A question of method or epistemology? *British Journal of Sociology, 35,* 75-92.

DeFriese, G. H., & Fielding, J. E. (1990). Health risk assessment and the clinical practice of preventive medicine. In R. B. Goldbloom & R. S. Lawrence (Eds.), *Preventing disease: Beyond the rhetoric* (pp. 460-466). New York: Springer-Verlag.

Engels, G. L. (1977). The need for a new medical model: The challenge for biomedicine. *Science, 196*, 129-136.

Epp, J. (1986). *Achieving health for all: A framework for health promotion*. Ottawa: Department of National Health and Welfare.

Evans, R. G., & Stoddart, G. L. (1990). Producing health, consuming health care. *Social Science and Medicine, 31*, 1347-1363.

Fishbein, M., & Ajzen, I. (1975). *Belief, attitude, intention and behavior: An introduction to theory and research*. Boston: Addison-Wesley.

Hanson, P. G. (1985). *The joy of stress*. Islington, Ontario: Hanson Stress Management Organization.

Jeffery, R. W. (1989). Risk behaviors and health: Contrasting individual and population perspectives. *American Psychologist, 44*, 1194-1202.

Lalonde, M. (1974). *A new perspective on the health of Canadians*. Ottawa: Department of National Health and Welfare.

Levin, L. S. (1987, Summer). Every silver lining has a cloud: The limits of health promotion. *Social Policy*, pp. 57-60.

Meehl, P. E. (1978). Theoretical risks and tabular asterisks: Sir Karl, Sir Ronald, and the slow progress of soft psychology. *Journal of Consulting and Clinical Psychology, 46*, 806-834.

Miller, J. G. (1978). *Living systems*. New York: McGraw-Hill.

Norman, R. (1986). *The nature and correlates of health behavior* (Health Promotion Series No. 2). Ottawa: Department of National Health and Welfare.

Phillips, D. C. (1987). *Philosophy, science and social inquiry*. New York: Pergamon.

Prochaska, J. O., & DiClemente, C. C. (1986). Toward a comprehensive model of change. In W. R. Miller & N. Heather (Eds.), *Treating addictive behaviors: Processes of change* (pp. 3-27). New York: Plenum.

Robbins, G., Powers, D., & Burgess, S. (1991). *A wellness way of life*. Dubuque, IA: William C Brown.

Roemer, M. I. (1984). The value of medical care for health promotion. *American Journal of Public Health, 74*, 243-248.

Rose, G. (1981). Strategy of prevention: Lessons from cardiovascular disease. *British Medical Journal, 282*, 1847-1851.

Russell, M. A. H., Wilson, C., Taylor, C., & Baker, C. D. (1979). Effect of general practitioner's advice against smoking. *British Medical Journal, 2*, 231-235.

Samuels, M., & Samuels, N. (1988). *The well audit*. New York: Summit.

Schunk, D. H., & Carbonari, J. P. (1984). Self-efficacy models. In J. D. Matarazzo, S. M. Weiss, J. A. Herd, N. E. Miller, & S. M. Weiss (Eds.), *Behavioral health: A handbook of health enhancement and disease prevention* (pp. 230-247). New York: John Wiley.

Schwenk, T. L., Clark, C. H., Jones, G. R., Simmons, R. C., & Coleman, M. L. (1982). Defining a behavioral science curriculum for family physicians: What do patients think? *Journal of Family Practice, 15*, 339-345.

Skinner, H. A. (1987). Self-report instruments for family assessment. In T. Jacob (Ed.), *Family interaction and psychopathology* (pp. 427-452). New York: Plenum.

Skinner, H. A., Holt, S., Sheu, W. J., & Israel, Y. (1986). Clinical versus laboratory detection of alcohol abuse: The Alcohol Clinical Index. *British Medical Journal, 292*, 1703-1708.

Sobal, J., Valente, C. M., Muncie, H. L., Levine, D. M., & Deforge, B. R. (1985). Physician's beliefs about the importance of 25 health promoting behaviors. *American Journal of Public Health, 75*, 1427-1428.

Steinhauer, P. D., Santa-Barbara, J., & Skinner, H. A. (1984). The process model of family functioning. *Canadian Journal of Psychiatry, 29*, 77-87.

Transport Canada. (1990). [Road safety leaflet TP2436]. Ottawa, Ontario: Author.

U.S. Department of Health and Human Resources. (1980). *Promoting health, preventing disease: Objectives for the nation.* Washington, DC: Government Printing Office.

U.S. Surgeon General. (1979). *Healthy people: The surgeon-general's report on health promotion and disease prevention* (DHEW Publication No. 7955071). Washington, DC: Department of Health, Education and Welfare.

Wallace, P. G., & Haines, A. P. (1984). General practitioner and health promotion: What patients think. *British Medical Journal, 289*, 534-536.

Wechsler, H., Levine, S., Idelson, R. K., Rohman, M., & Taylor, J. O. (1983). The physician's role in health promotion: A survey of primary-care practitioners. *New England Journal of Medicine, 308*, 97-100.

Weiss, S. M. (1984). Health hazard/health risk appraisals. In J. D. Matarazzo, S. M. Weiss, J. A. Herd, N. E. Miller, & S. M. Weiss (Eds.), *Behavioral health: A handbook of health enhancement and disease prevention* (pp. 275-294). New York: John Wiley.

World Health Organization. (1978). *Declaration of Alma Ata.* Geneva: World Health Organization.

World Health Organization. (1986). *Ottawa charter for health promotion.* Geneva: World Health Organization.

14 Assessment of an Intervention in Primary Care: Counseling Patients on Smoking Cessation

DOUGLAS M. C. WILSON

When assessing the success of any intervention, it is useful to distinguish between *efficacy* and *effectiveness*. The former refers to whether the intervention works under relatively ideal, controlled research conditions, whereas the latter refers to how well it works under more typical "real-world" conditions. Research that evaluates the success of physicians in counseling their patients who smoke to quit shows that these professionals can be efficacious with relatively brief interventions (Kottke, Battista, DeFriese, & Brekke, 1988; Ockene, 1987; Pederson, 1984). It is not clear, however, to what extent or under what circumstances they are effective in routine practice.

Primary care physicians are in an ideal position to deliver this type of counseling, as up to 70% of the adult population sees a physician during any one year (Rowmer, 1984); thus it is important to assess their impact and role from a population health perspective. What factors determine the impact of physician counseling in clinical practice?

Traditional medical education has not generally included training in how to help patients change their living patterns. There is an obvious need then to make such training available to practicing physicians through continuing medical education (CME).

139

Yet what do we know about changing clinical practices through CME? Several comprehensive reviews in the past 10 years (Abrahamson, 1984; Bertram & Brooks-Bertram, 1980; Segall et al., 1981) have examined the degree of experimental rigor exhibited in the design of CME-sponsored interventions and, for those meeting design criteria, summarized their impact on (a) physician knowledge, attitudes, and behavior and (b) patient outcomes. Their findings have indicated that few studies measured physician behavior, and still fewer assessed patient outcomes. In a review by Haynes, Davis, McKibbon, and Tugwell (1984), only 7 of 248 CME studies investigated met the criteria for rigorous design; of these 7, all reported significant changes in physician performance, but only 3 assessed patient outcomes, and only 1 of these demonstrated improvement. Haynes et al. conclude that change in practitioner behavior "seems to bear a relationship to the intensity of the intervention" and that "more complex educational strategies resulted in more consistent and substantial effects." Education research suggests that changes in physician clinical behavior will be more likely to occur when educational planners build in strategies such as cuing, modeling, and reinforcement (Bandura, 1977; Haynes, Taylor, & Sackett, 1979).

It therefore became clear that studies of education interventions of physicians to change their clinical behavior with respect to smoking cessation should be done. In the study reported here, we compared smoking cessation rates between the patients of one group of physicians who provided only their usual care for smokers; a second group, who were asked to provide advice and an offer of nicotine gum; and a third group who received special training in dealing with this issue.

Methods

Using an Ontario Medical Association listing, we contacted 460 family physicians practicing within a 40-mile radius of the research center, asking them to participate in the study. Of the 102 who responded positively, 12 withdrew or were set aside prior to randomization and 7 after it. The remaining 83 physicians, representing 70 practices, were randomly allocated by practice to the three treatment groups. Comparison of the dropouts and the participants revealed no significant differences that might have biased the composition of the experimental groups.

Smoking patients were recruited for the study by the office receptionist when they visited their physician for a routine appointment. Our intention was to recruit as representative a sample as possible; thus receptionists were asked to follow a standardized protocol, asking each eligible smoker to participate until a maximum of two each day agreed. A total of 1,942 patients were recruited in this way. Along with completing a questionnaire, patients were asked to sign a consent letter that stated that they agreed to be followed and emphasized that they were not necessarily agreeing to try to stop smoking. "Exit interviews" consisted of phone interviews of patients from all groups within 3 days of their first visit to the physician. Open-ended questions assessed the content of their visit with regard to smoking cessation.

DESIGN

They also agreed to complete a follow-up questionnaire and a saliva validation test one year later, to assess outcome. The experimental variation in condition began when the patient went in to see the physician. In Condition 1 (Usual Care), the physicians were not to know which of their patients had agreed to participate in the study. If it was part of their usual practice to address the issue of a patient smoking, this occurred; otherwise, it did not. In Condition 2 (Gum Only), the physicians were cued by a project document indicating the patient's agreement to participate and were instructed simply (a) to advise that patient to quit smoking and (b) to offer nicotine gum as an aid to quitting. In Condition 3 (Gum Plus), physicians received premailed background reading, attended a four-hour training session, and were given print materials for office and patient use. The maneuver they were requested to apply comprised six components: challenging the patient to quit; negotiation of a target date; offer of Nicorette (a prescription nicotine-bearing chewing gum designed as a cessation adjunct to reduce withdrawal symptoms); a written contract to formalize patient decisions on these first three components; provision of a sheet of "Quit Tips" to be posted on the home refrigerator, outlining behavioral self-management tactics; and the offer of up to five follow-up supportive visits. A project flow sheet cued these physicians as to which patients were in the study, and it also helped them to remember the ingredients of the intervention.

In the training session, the obstacles that busy family practitioners state get in the way of dealing with patients who smoke were addressed. First, many physicians are pessimistic about whether people are able to change, based on discouraging results from previous attempts to encourage smokers, alcoholics, or sedentary or obese individuals to change their life-styles. Second, physicians often feel a lack of confidence in their effectiveness in counseling and as change agents and feel that they have had little or no training or modeling of skills in dealing with cigarette smoking issues. Third, many feel that dealing with issues of health promotion is a very time-consuming process and, because of their already busy practices, they are unable to find the time to do so. Fourth, some consider life-style to be a matter of personal choice and feel that they should not be "preaching" at their patients regarding how they choose to live. Finally, there does not seem to be a recognized fee for dealing with this type of health problem in an ongoing way.

The recruited physicians indicated that they would like to be trained in an effective method that had already been tested and that preferably fit the medical model. They also insisted that the intervention be very simple so that it could be easily remembered. As well, it was important that the initial contact not consume more than 5 minutes, because it would usually be added onto a regularly scheduled office visit. Finally, as with other health maintenance issues, the physicians felt that they would be more likely to perform the intervention if they had a reminder system.

Outcomes

PHYSICIAN COMPLIANCE

The results of the exit interviews are shown in Table 14.1. All differences recorded were in the expected direction, with Gum Plus physicians more likely to exhibit the procedures they were trained to follow (such as offering advice, inviting patients back for follow-up, and providing take-home materials) compared with physicians in the other two groups. Physicians in the Gum Only group did suggest using gum to their patients nearly as often as did the Gum

Table 14.1 Initial Visit Exit Interview

Actions of Doctor Toward Patient	Usual Care (n = 90)	Gum Only (n = 94)	Gum Plus (Training) (n = 96)	p	χ^2
Raised subject of smoking	31.1	70.2	85.4	< .001	61.96
Suggested quitting	24.4	64.0	84.4	< .001	59.72
Offered help	12.2	61.7	84.5	< .001	106.93
Suggested gum method	8.9	58.5	62.5	< .001	38.15
Asked for quit date	2.2	11.7	54.2	< .001	80.84
Suggested follow-up visit	4.4	22.3	83.3	< .001	137.22
Gave reading material	2.0	17.0	80.2	< .001	144.07

NOTE: χ^2 values are based on differences among the three groups.

Plus physicians but had lower rates for all the other intervention behaviors.

PATIENT OUTCOMES

Patients were considered to be successful quitters if, on the one-year questionnaire,

(a) they reported not having smoked even one puff of a cigarette in the last week;
(b) they reported not smoking a pipe or cigar or using chewing tobacco; and
(c) a biochemical validation test produced a saliva continine value of less than or equal to 10 ng/l, or a saliva thiocyanate level of less than 1,724 umol/l (100 ug/ml) if the patients were still using nicotine gum.

The unit of randomization in this study was the clinical practice. Therefore, although patient smoking cessation is the primary outcome, the appropriate analysis requires the use of a single outcome measure for each of the 70 practices. The proportion of patients who met our definition of success in each practice (the practice quit rate) was therefore used as the outcome for each practice. Self-reported cessation rates were adjusted after biochemical validation by saliva continine analysis.

Using 3-month sustained abstinence as the primary outcome, adjusted cessation rates were 4.4%, 6.1%, and 8.8% in the Usual Care, Gum Only, and Gum Plus groups, respectively. In terms of the individual comparisons, there was clearly no difference between Usual Care and Gum only; therefore, it was deemed appropriate to collapse these two conditions and together compare them with Gum Plus. Again, for 3-month sustained abstinence, the Gum Plus condition was found to be superior to the other two treatments.

Discussion

The results indicate that the physician training procedure described here produced higher cessation rates among smoking patients than either usual care only or usual care and an offer of nicotine gum. Relative to the Usual Care group, the Gum Plus intervention produced a 100% increase in biochemically validated smoking cessation: 8.8% versus 4.4%. In absolute terms, this increase could be viewed as having limited clinical significance; however, viewed on a population- or communitywide basis, it is potentially important.

Simple advice to quit seems to stimulate patients to at least attempt to stop smoking. Therefore, the training of physicians on a large scale should first motivate them to address cessation with all of their smoking patients who have any interest in stopping. Second, continuing education should provide knowledge and skills that will help physicians became more effective providers of cessation interventions.

Clinicians may not be impressed with the cessation rates produced through this intervention. When they consider the numbers of smokers in their practices, however, the actual number of potential ex-smokers is substantial. It is this access to smokers and the opportunity for repeated efforts to help them that makes the potential of physicians' interventions important.

References

Abrahamson, S. (1984). Evaluation of continuing education in the health professions: The state of the art. *Evaluation and the Health Professions, 7*(1), 3-24.

Bandura, A. (1977). *Social learning theory.* Englewood Cliffs, NJ: Prentice-Hall.

Bertram, D. A., & Brooks-Bertram, P. A. (1980). The evaluation of continuing medical education: A literature review. *Health Education Monographs, 5*(4), 282-288.

Haynes, R. B., Davis, D. A., McKibbon, A., & Tugwell, P. (1984). A critical appraisal of the efficacy of continuing medical education. *Journal of the American Medical Association, 251,* 61-64.

Haynes, R. B., Taylor, D. W., & Sackett, D. L. (Eds.). (1979). *Compliance in health care.* Baltimore, MD: Johns Hopkins University Press.

Kottke, T. E., Battista, R. N., DeFriese, G. H., & Brekke, M. L. (1988). Attributes of successful smoking cessation intervention in medical practice: A meta-analysis of 39 controlled trials. *Journal of the American Medical Association, 259,* 2883-2889.

Ockene, J. K. (1987). Physician-delivered interventions for smoking cessation: Strategies for increasing effectiveness. *Preventive Medicine, 16,* 723-737.

Pederson, L. L. (1984). Role of the physician in smoking cessation. In U.S. Department of Health and Human Services, *Health consequences of smoking for chronic obstructive lung disease: A report of the surgeon-general* (DHHS Publication No. [PHS] 84-50205). Washington, DC: Government Printing Office.

Rowmer, M. I. (1984). The value of medical care for health promotion. *American Journal of Public Health, 74,* 243-248.

Segall, A., Barker, W. H., Cobb, S., Jackson, G., Noen, J., Shindell, S., Stokes, J., & Ericsson, S. (1981). Development of a competency-based approach to teaching preventive medicine. *Preventive Medicine, 10,* 726-735.

15 Assessing Primary Health
   Care Delivery

J. IVAN WILLIAMS

A major objective of health policy is the availability and accessibility of primary health care. Health policy planners in the United States continue to look at the Canadian model for national health insurance as one means for ensuring primary health care. There have been numerous attempts to improve primary health care in the United States and Canada through extended health insurance plans, increased numbers of physicians, and the organization of medical practice. In this chapter, I review selected studies on particular models and issues in primary health care delivery in the United States and Canada. The goal is to develop an overall perspective on the current state of primary medical care in Canada as it has evolved since the introduction of national health insurance in 1969.

The Tasks of Primary Health
Care Delivery

Parker (1974) defined the tasks of primary health care agencies as follows:

1. They serve as the entry, screening, and referral point for personal health care.
2. They provide a full range of basic health care services.

3. They provide stabilizing support for patients and families in times of trouble or crises.
4. They assume responsibility for the continuing management and coordination of personal health care services throughout the entire care process.

On the basis of this definition, Parker found primary health care in the United States to be lacking in terms of the number of providers, the fragmentation of services across specialties, the organization of practices, the availability and accessibility of services, and coverage of costs for consumers.

In the 1970s, a series of conferences were held on the American and Canadian health care sectors (LeClair, 1975), with the innovations in Quebec being a particular object of study (Castonguay, 1975). Years later, the problems in health care policy in the United States continue to mount. A consideration of its average annual health care expenditures per capita in 1985 is instructive: $2,230 (in Canadian dollars) compared with about $1,570 in Canada (Health and Welfare Canada, 1987). Public health dollars covered about 55% of these costs, compared with 75% in Canada.

The only category of expenditures per capita that was higher for Canada was drugs: $169 as compared with $140 for the United States. (This is one of the unique features of health care in Canada. Not only are the average expenditures on drugs in Canada among the highest for the 24 countries that are members of the Organisation for Economic Co-operation and Development (OECD), but the rate of increase over the past decade is comparatively high as well [Schieber, 1987].)

For the category "Other Costs" that includes the costs for prepayment administration, public health, capital expenditures, health research, and miscellaneous health costs, the average per capita expenditure was $484 in the United States as compared with $225 in Canada. Included in these figures are the costs for administering health care. In 1960, about 5% of the GNP was expended on health care in Canada; this figure was slightly higher for the United States. The costs of health care administration were between 0.15% and 0.20% of the GNP for both countries in that year. By 1987, the United States was expending 11% of its GNP on health care, and the administrative costs had climbed to about 0.55% of the GNP, or about 5% of the total costs of health care. During the same period in Canada, the expenditure on health care increased to 9% of the GNP, but the share of the GNP going to administration declined to about 0.10%, or about 1.1% of the total costs of health care (Evans, Barer, & Hertzman, 1991). The layered systems for providing, managing, and financing health services in the United States are extraordinarily expensive.

Physician Services

During the first half of this century, the number of physicians in Canada increased from about 5,000 in 1901 to 12,000 in 1951. Before World War II, this increase failed to keep pace with the growth of the population, and the failure would have been dramatic had it not been for the net migration of physicians from other countries, principally the United Kingdom (Judek, 1964).

Following the report from the Royal Commission on Health Services (1964), four strategies were employed to increase the number of health professionals, particularly general practitioners. These were the development of four new medical schools and enlarging the class sizes of the existing ones; encouraging the immigration of physicians and discouraging their emigration to the United States; expanding the roles of nurses in the provision of primary care; and promoting Community Health Centers for the reorganization of primary health care (Williams, 1981).

Between 1951 and 1988, the number of physicians increased from 12,000 to about 58,000, more than doubling the ratio from about 10 to 22 per 10,000 population. Even so, a third of all physicians are graduates of foreign medical schools. (Controls are now in place to severely limit the number of physicians admitted from other countries and licensed to practice.)

In 1962, the College of General Practice changed its name to the College of Family Physicians of Canada (CFPC) and refocused on the development of undergraduate and postgraduate training programs in family medicine, while maintaining an emphasis on continuing medical education. By 1975, all 16 medical schools had undergraduate and residency training programs in family medicine. The percentage of graduating students entering general or family practice increased, so that, by 1988, more than half of the physicians in active practice were providing primary medical care;

40% of these were members of the CFPC, and 70% of the members were certificated in the discipline (College of Family Physicians of Canada, personal communication, 1991). Borgiel and his colleagues (1989) were among the first to demonstrate convincingly that the graduates of family medicine residency programs provide a higher quality of care than other family physicians. Quebec became the first province to require certification by the CFPC of all new graduates wishing to provide primary care.

For the most part, the availability of primary care physicians in Canada is assured except for remote rural areas, where provinces continue to have difficulty in recruiting physicians to practice despite a wide range of incentives. It is now evident that increasing the number of physicians does not ensure equal access in all regions.

Commissions, inquiries, and task forces at the federal and provincial levels have studied the "surplus" of physicians. Provinces tightly control the numbers of immigrating physicians who intend to practice as well as the number of postgraduate residency positions that they will fund. Quebec has already required a reduction in the class sizes of medical schools, and other provinces will likely follow.

No self-respecting medical professional association has ever admitted to a surplus of physicians, even though there is agreement with the policies restricting immigration. The professional bodies hold that numbers of physicians should keep pace with increase in demands for services, particularly as the population of Canada is aging.

Evans, Roch, and Pascoe (1987) studied the effects of the physician supply increase on the costs of medical services in Manitoba. In 1981, there were 16.1 physicians per 10,000 residents of Manitoba, an increase of 29% since 1971. In terms of constant dollars adjusted for inflation, the average billings per general practitioner in 1981 were $86,054 (a 3% increase) and $105,931 for specialists (an increase of 0.2%). The billings per capita in 1981 were $131, an increase of 30%. During 1981, 87% of Manitoba residents saw a physician for at least one visit, an increase of 7% over the earlier time period.

Evans et al. focused on the impact of the increase of GPs in Winnipeg, where the number went from 4.2 per 10,000 in 1971 to 6.3 in 1981. GPs in solo practice increased by 100, while there was

Table 15.1 Changes in General Practitioner Activities in Winnipeg by Solo and Group Practice, 1971/1972 to 1981/1982

Activities	Solo Practice Amount	Change % 1971	Group Practice Amount	Change % 1971
General practitioner activities:				
GPs per 10,000 population	4.4	+99.6	1.9	+4.0
apparent patients per GP	1,732	+6.5	2,017	−8.7
contacts per patients	2.7	−9.3	2.8	26.5
billings per patient contact	$15.60	−6.7	$15.33	−8.6
annual billings per GP	$74,047	−9.9	$87,211	5.5
Patient sharing activities:				
patient multiplier—other MDs seen per GP patient	3.8	62.9	3.5	15.7
revenue multiplier for MDs— other MD fees per GP billing	4.8	96.7	4.2	1.4

SOURCE: Adapted from Evans et al. (1987, 1991).
NOTE: All dollar amounts are in constant dollars.

minimal change in the number in group practice (see Table 15.1). The average number of "apparent patients" per GP—patients who come to a practice in a given year—increased for those in solo practice and declined for those in group practice. The contacts per patient declined by 9% over the decade for GPs in solo practice but increased by 27% for those in group practice. For both groups, the billings per patient contact declined. The net result was that the average annual billings of GPs in solo practice ($74,047) represented a 10% decline in constant dollars over the decade, while those of GPs in group practice ($87,211) went up by 6%.

It should be noted that these investigators did not adjust for years in practice. A new physician, particularly in a city, takes 3 to 5 years to develop a practice and reach full earning power. The reduced level of billing activity of GPs reflects in part the large influx of new graduates into practice.

The next step in the analysis was to look at the use of medical services from the perspective of the patients. Table 15.1 shows that, on average, each patient of a GP in solo practice saw 3.8 other physicians in 1981, a slightly higher multiplying effect than for patients of GPs in group practice (3.5).

The result was to multiply billings for physicians. Other physicians billed 4.8 dollars for every dollar billed by a solo GP, and 4.2 dollars for every dollar billed by a GP in group practice. The revenue multiplier for patients of solo GPs in 1981 had doubled since 1971. About 25% of the revenues went to other GPs who were networked with the base physicians and shared their patients, while the remainder went to specialists.

The patterns of revenue-multiplying for patients of GPs in group practice changed relatively little from 1971 to 1981; as the average number of patients per physician declined, physicians in general and solo GPs in particular generated more services per patient visit and ensured additional fees for other physicians by increasing the rate by which they passed their patients through a referral network. The average income of physicians kept pace with the cost of living during the 10-year interval, despite the 29% increase in the supply of physicians.

Fuchs and Hahn (1990) compared expenditures on physician services in Manitoba and Iowa. In 1985 U.S. dollars, the fees for procedures in Iowa were twice as high as the comparable fees in Manitoba, but the net income of physicians in Iowa was only 60% higher. There were two reasons for this. The overhead costs in Iowa were higher than in Manitoba, so physicians there kept less of their earnings. Furthermore, physicians in Manitoba provided 45% more services per capita than those in Iowa. American physicians rely on high fees to maintain their incomes; Canadians maintain theirs by increased billings.

There has been a marked increase in the enrollment of women in Canadian medical schools. In the 1960s, about 10% of the graduates of medical schools were women (Ryten, 1988). By 1988, women made up 40% of the classes in medicine. Women are more likely to become family physicians than men. There are questions as to whether the patterns and style of practice for women are markedly different than those of men and, if so, what the implications are for the delivery of primary care.

At McMaster University, there is a group of researchers who have been undertaking a series of studies to determine whether graduates of the "new" medical school practice medicine differently than graduates of "traditional" medical school. The medical school at McMaster has a 3-year curriculum based on problem solving and small group teaching. Keane, Woodward, Ferrier,

Table 15.2 Characteristics of Primary Care Physicians by Sex

Characteristics of Physicians	Men %	Women %
McMaster graduates	50	50
Graduated before 1980	57	27*
In full-time practice	89	68*
Certificated by CFPC	36	54*
Practice in urban setting	89	86

SOURCE: Adapted from Keane et al. (1990).
*p < .01.

Cohen, and Goldsmith (1990) studied the billing practices of primary care physicians in Ontario, focusing on 212 women and 432 men who graduated from McMaster University between 1972 and 1983 and an equal number of graduates from other medical schools in Ontario for the same years. The characteristics of these physicians by sex are displayed in Table 15.2. Comparatively speaking, the women were more likely to have graduated after 1979, to be in part-time practice (averaging less than $6,000 in monthly Ontario Health Insurance Plan [OHIP] billings), and to be certificated by the CFPC.

As shown in Table 15.3, male doctors generated more earnings by seeing more patients; however, while women saw fewer patients, they generated more services per patient visit, hence their OHIP billings per patient were higher. This finding is consistent with the general observation that women in practice tend to spend more time with individual patients than their male counterparts. The average woman in practice provides about 60% of the medical services of the average man. The implication of this is that 167 women would have to be trained to practice medicine to equal the productivity of the 100 male physicians.

Gender has proven to be a far more important determinant of style of practice than place of graduation.

Community Health Centers

Currently in Canada, family physicians work in environments as diverse as private practice, emergency departments of hospitals,

Table 15.3 Average OHIP Billings by Sex of Primary Care Physicians

OHIP Monthly Billings	Men	Women
Active months of practice	11.6	10.9
Services provided	775	452**
OHIP earnings	$12,644	$7,741**
Patients seen	394	242*
Services per patient	2.1	2.3
Billings per patient	$36.99	$45.99*

SOURCE: Adapted from Keane et al. (1990).
*0.01 < p < 0.05.
**p < .01.

acute care and chronic care hospitals, nursing homes, sports clinics, walk-in clinics, occupational health departments, and hospice centers. Considerable time, energy, and attention have been given to the definition of the optimal practice arrangements. In 1973, a federal-provincial task force recommended the creation of community health centers, the employment of teams of salaried, primary health care professionals, a flexible and innovative use of the personnel, a range of health promotion and prevention services, and improved access to care in terms of location, hours of operation, and focus on groups with special needs (Health and Welfare Canada, 1973).

Derivations of the concept can be found in the Centres Locaux de Services Communautaires (CLSCs) in Quebec, Health Services Organizations (HSOs) and Community Health Centres (CHCs) in Ontario, and Community Health Centres in Saskatchewan. Some early studies of the centers in Saskatchewan (Anderson & Crichton, 1973; Wolfe & Badgley, 1973) suggested they provided comprehensive services at lower costs. While the costs of primary health care are comparable to or greater than those of fee-for-service practice, comprehensive services in the CHCs have led to reductions in hospital admissions for investigative work-ups. Barer (1981) used simulation models to estimate the savings in health care dollars that could be achieved in Canada if all primary care were provided through the CHCs.

Subsequent reviews of the HSOs and CHCs in Ontario and the CLSCs in Quebec indicated that these centers provide services to fewer than 5% of residents. The organizations became embodiments of the values and beliefs of the reform-minded health professionals who staffed them and became unresponsive to the mandates set forth by the governments in the two provinces (Hastings & Vayda, 1986). The governments have since revamped their programs, and Quebec has issued a new mandate for the CLSCs to fulfill. Both governments are exploring model comprehensive health organizations for the provision of integrated primary health care and hospital services, along the lines of the original model of Health Maintenance Organizations (HMOs) in the United States.

In the United States, HMOs and private groups of physicians compete for prepaid, contractual arrangements with employers and third parties who provide health insurance and pay for the services. HMOs grew rapidly throughout the 1960s and 1970s, and by 1989 32.5 million Americans were enrolled for their services. Their growth has now slowed and they have been criticized for unduly rationing care to the point of compromising quality to control costs. They have also been criticized for enrolling only younger and healthier individuals, whose needs for health care are relatively low. The major consumer complaints focus on the lack of a personal physician and the overall impersonal quality of care.

Payments and Outcomes

Both those who manage and those who pay for health care are under pressure to find methods and mechanisms demonstrating the cost-effectiveness of the services they provide. There are few studies that relate the outcomes of the various organizational arrangements and payment mechanisms for primary health care.

The best known study is the Rand Health Insurance Experiment, which involved the random assignment of 7,699 persons from 6 American cities to 1 of 14 fee-for-service health insurance plans. These individuals were followed for 3 to 5 years, and 86% completed all phases of the study. The research team developed and employed a broad range of cost, process, and outcome measures to assess the impact of copayments by the consumer on the uses of services, the quality of care, and health-related outcomes (Brook et al., 1983; Brook et al., 1990).

Process and outcome criteria for quality of care were developed for 13 adult and 5 child chronic conditions. Health status measures for physical functioning, role functioning, mental health, social contacts, and general health perceptions were completed both at the beginning and at the end of the study. The research team collected additional information on health habits such as smoking, and physiological measures, such as blood pressure, weight, serum cholesterol, and vision. One key outcome was to determine whether variations in care would alter the risk of death.

Literally hundreds of publications have been written about the Rand study: its design, the development of its methods, its payment plans, and the relationships between copayments, process, and outcomes. The key findings compared persons who received their care free of payment against those who had to share in the costs.

Persons receiving free care made more visits for health care, and their costs were one-third higher than those of the individuals who shared costs. With respect to outcomes, the persons receiving free care had better vision at the end of the study, and low-income participants receiving free care had better hypertension control and a lower risk of dying compared with low-income individuals in cost-sharing plans. Overall, the quality of care for chronic conditions was high: 80% of the criteria for the specified conditions were met across the various plans.

In a side study, an additional 775 adults were randomized to an HMO in Seattle. Compared with the HMO participants, fee-for-service individuals had lower rates of hospital admissions and were less satisfied with their care. Provider compliance in the HMO with the process and outcome criteria for chronic conditions was better. With respect to overall outcomes, there were paradoxical findings: Lower-income participants in HMOs did worse than their fee-for-service counterparts, while higher-income participants did better (Ware, Brook, & Rogers, 1986). The findings gave substance to the prevailing criticisms of the HMOs.

Wagner and Bledsoe (1990) queried the failure to use a concurrent control group of patients enrolled in the HMO in the Seattle portion of the study. They defined such a group and reevaluated the comparisons. While these authors agree that the HMO participants were less satisfied with the care they received, they believe the adverse results attributed to HMOs were more likely artifacts of the methods of the study than indicative of true differences. They questioned the suitability of the Rand methods, particularly outcome measures, for judging the benefits and effects of the delivery of primary care.

The limitations of the Rand study should be noted. Although its participants came from a broad range of income groupings, it excluded both very poor families, particularly those living in the core of central cities, and high-income families as well as elderly individuals and persons with chronic illnesses and disabling conditions. Thus its results cannot be generalized to those individuals most likely to benefit from free care.

The contributions of the Rand research team in developing process and outcome health measures are widely acknowledged. The ability of these methods to detect significant changes in health status over time, particularly over a 3- to 5-year time period, however, remains an open question. On the whole, the methods for assessing the process and outcomes of care for children were far less satisfactory than were the measures of adult health.

It appears that certain beliefs on the part of the physician can affect costs. Wright and Kane (1982) asked family physicians to predict whether their patients would have poor or good outcomes and followed 1,757 patients to determine the accuracy of these prognoses. Accuracy proved to be low: The physicians predicted that 6% of the patients would do poorly whereas in fact 24% of them actually did, while 43% of those given a poor prognosis actually did well. Regardless of the actual outcomes, the average costs of care were 50% higher for the group with poor prognoses ($30) than for those with good ones ($20). When comparing those who actually had bad outcomes against those with good outcomes, the average cost was only marginally higher ($23 versus $20). Thus a prediction of poor prognosis on the part of the physician led to higher costs, even when the prediction was wrong.

Bass and his colleagues (1986) examined the predictors of early resolution of presenting problems for 232 patients presenting with new episodes of abdominal complaints, back or neck pain, chest pain, fatigue, headache, eye problems, or rectal bleeding. Working with physicians in 23 family practices, they asked physicians to predict whether the problems would have early or late resolution. Patients predicted to have early resolutions were interviewed by telephone at 1 month, and those with the prognosis of late resolution were interviewed at 3 months. The results of these interviews were matched with the process of care charted in the records.

The best predictors of early resolution of symptoms were that (a) patient agreed with the doctor's assessment of the problem, (b) patient reported no stress, (c) psychosocial factors were recorded on the chart, (d) the symptoms had been present for less than 2 weeks before the visit, and (e) the patient had seen the physician within the past year for other care. The best predictors of late resolution were (a) complaints of chest pain, rectal bleeding, abdominal pain, or headache; (b) failure of the patient to discuss his or her problem with others; and (c) notes in the patient's chart to the effect that the physician thought counseling was required.

It is interesting to note that, apart from the type of presenting problem, the timing of resolution appears to be strongly related to the dynamics of the doctor-patient relationship. Patients do better when the problem is discussed and understood and when consideration is given to psychosocial factors.

It is extraordinarily difficult to relate the patterns of primary care to outcomes and to estimate the cost-effectiveness of different patterns of care. Beyond the problems of measuring outcomes, there are marked variations in resource use, no small part of which occur by chance. Moreover, the linkage of health services to outcomes has to take into account the compliance of both providers and consumers, the severity of the presenting problem, and the presence of systemic illnesses that compromise the response to therapy. Nevertheless, there are now two major efforts under way to measure these relationships.

InterStudy is a voluntary association of prepaid practice arrangements under the leadership of Paul Ellwood, the "godfather" of HMOs. Ellwood has commissioned teams of researchers to generate generic measures of health status as well as disease-specific measures. These include a 36-item questionnaire for measuring functional status and quality of life (Ware, 1989) and disease-specific instruments called TyPEs (Technology of Patient Experiences) to examine alcohol abuse, asthma, cataracts, chronic obstructive lung disease, coronary artery disease, depression, gall-bladder disease, low back pain, osteoporosis, and prostatism. Tools for other diseases are being constructed as well.

The Agency for Health Policy and Research (AHCPR) in the United States has contracted Patient Outcome Research Teams (PORTs) to develop outcome measures that can be used to assess the quality and effectiveness of medical care for acute myocardial infarction, back pain, cataract management, prostate disease, and total knee replacement (Salive, Mayfield, & Weissman, 1990). The teams are to base their measures on meta-analyses of the literature; analyses of claims data, surveys, cohort studies, and intervention studies; and decision analysis.

Eddy and Billings (1988) enter a note of caution about the state of knowledge in medical science, noting that, for most health problems, we lack scientific evidence on achievable outcomes. The following areas should be considered:

(a) the financing of outcome-measuring activities;

(b) the development of information-management systems to assure that the requisite data are maintained in standard form suitable for analysis;

(c) determining who will do the counting and who will be held accountable for the results;

(d) defining the appropriate unit for analysis and management (the individual provider, group practice or hospital, county/district/ region, province/state, or the nation as a whole); and

(e) assuring that the results will be translated into management practices or payment mechanisms for correcting the problems.

It will take some time to translate these methods into tools that can be used in the management and financing of health care.

On Getting Here from There

There is continued interest in the United States in adapting the model of medical care insurance in Canada for the financing and management of Medicare (Naylor, 1991). It is reasonable to ask, then: What changes have occurred in primary health care delivery in Canada since the introduction of publicly funded, universal medical care insurance? The following checklist may help in formulating an answer to this question:

Primary Health Care Delivery	*Result*
Supply of providers	Increased
Types of practices	Diversified
Consumer contacts	Increased
Services per contact	Increased
Costs of services	Increased
One source for primary contact	Decreased
Continuity, coordination of care	Decreased
Overall quality of care	???

In Canada, health care policy has led to an increase in the number of providers and the availability of care. Providers in return have diversified their activities and are generating services at a rate in excess of the growth of the population or of changes in the demonstrable needs for health care. The proliferation of primary care and the generation of medical care services have taken precedence over the coordination and control of comprehensive services in the management of consumer problems. To this extent, there has been an abdication of responsibility for the tasks of primary health care delivery.

To conclude, the availability and accessibility of primary care physicians have increased, and these physicians are maintaining their average earnings by increasing the number and range of services they provide. They have done so while abrogating their responsibilities for tasks of comprehensive, continuous, and coordinated care. New strategies are required to accomplish the tasks of primary care while controlling the costs and uses of health care services.

References

Anderson, D. O., & Crichton, A. O. J. (1973). *What price group practice: A study of charges and expenditures for medical care.* Vancouver: University of British Columbia, Health Sciences Centre.

Barer, M. L. (1981). *Community health centres and hospital costs in Ontario.* Toronto: Ontario Economic Council.

Bass, M. J., Buck, C., Turner, L., Dickie, G., Pratt, G., & Robinson, H. C. (1986). The physician's actions and the outcome of illness in family practice. *Journal of Family Practice, 23,* 43-47.

Borgiel, A. E. M., Williams, J. I., Bass, M. J., Dunn, E. V., Evenson, M. K., Lamont, C. T., MacDonald, P. J., McCoy, J. M., & Spasoff, R. A. (1989). Quality of care in family practice: Does residency training make a difference? *Canadian Medical Association Journal, 140,* 1035-1043.

Brook, R. H., Kamberg, C. J., Lohr, K. N., Goldberg, G. A., Keeler, E. B., & Newhouse, J. P. (1990). Quality of ambulatory care: Epidemiology by insurance status and income. *Medical Care, 28,* 392-433.

Brook, R. H., Ware, J. E., Jr., Rogers, W. H., Keeler, E. M., Davies, A. R., Donald, C. A., Goldberg, G. A., Lohr, K. N., Masthay, P. C., & Newhouse, J. P. (1983). Does free care improve adults' health? Results from a randomized controlled trial. *New England Journal of Medicine, 309,* 1426-1434.

Castonguay, C. (1975). The Quebec experience: Effects on accessibility. In S. Andreopoulos (Ed.), *National health insurance: Can we learn from Canada?* (pp. 97-121). New York: John Wiley.

Eddy, D. M., & Billings, J. (1988). The quality of the medical evidence: Implications for quality of care. *Health Affairs, 7,* 19-32.

Evans, R. G., Barer, M. L., & Hertzman, C. (1991). The 20-year experiment: Accounting for, explaining, and evaluating health care cost containment in Canada and the United States. *Annual Review of Public Health, 12,* 482-518.

Evans, R. G., Roch, D. J., & Pascoe, D. W. (1987). Defensive reticulation: Physician supply increases and practice pattern changes in Manitoba, 1971 to 1981. In J. M. Horne (Ed.), *Proceedings of the Third Canadian Conference on Health Economics* (pp. 91-126). Winnipeg: University of Manitoba, Department of Social and Preventive Medicine.

Fuchs, V. R., & Hahn, J. S. (1990). How does Canada do it? A comparison of expenditures for physicians' services in the United States and Canada. *New England Journal of Medicine, 323,* 884-890.

Hastings, J. E. F., & Vayda, E. (1986). Health services organization and delivery: Promise and reality. In R. G. Evans & G. L. Stoddart (Eds.), *Medicare at maturity: Achievements, lessons, and challenges.* Calgary, Alberta: University of Calgary Press.

Health and Welfare Canada. (1973). *The community health centre in Canada: Vols. 1-3. Report of the community health centre project to the health minister.* Ottawa: Information Canada.

Health and Welfare Canada. (1987). *National health expenditures in Canada 1975-1985.* Ottawa: Minister of Supply and Services Canada.

Judek, S. (1964). *Medical manpower in Canada: A report to the Royal Commission on Health Services.* Ottawa: Queen's Printer.

Keane, D., Woodward, C. A., Ferrier, B. M., Cohen, M., & Goldsmith, C. H. (1990). Female and male physicians: Different practice profiles. *Canadian Family Physician, 37,* 72-81.

LeClair, M. (1975). The Canadian health care system. In S. Andreopoulos (Ed.), *National health insurance: Can we learn from Canada?* (pp. 11-92). New York: John Wiley.

Parker, A. W. (1974). The dimensions of primary care: Blueprints for change. In S. Andreopoulos (Ed.), *Primary care: Where medicine fails* (pp. 15-76). New York: John Wiley.

Naylor, C. D. (1991). The Canadian health care system: An overview and some comparisons with America. *Current Surgery, 48*(2), 115-122.

Ryten, E. (1988). The changing demographics of physician supply in Canada. In M. Watanbee (Ed.), *Physician manpower in Canada: Proceedings of the First and*

Second Annual Physician Manpower Conference (pp. 116-139). Ottawa: Association of Canadian Medical Colleges.

Salive, M. E., Mayfield, J. A., & Weissman, N. W. (1990). Patient outcomes research teams and the agency for health care policy and research. *Health Services Research, 25,* 697-708.

Schieber, G. J. (1987). *Financing and delivering health care: A comparative analysis of OECD countries* (Social Policies Studies No. 4). Paris: OECD.

Wagner, E. H., & Bledsoe, T. (1990). The Rand Health Insurance Experiment and HMOs. *Medical Care, 28,* 191-200.

Ware, J. E., Jr. (1989). *Health status questionnaire.* Boston: Quality Quest.

Ware, J. E., Jr., Brook, R. H., & Rogers, W. H. (1986). Comparisons of health outcomes at a health maintenance organization with those of fee-for-service care. *Lancet, 1,* 1017-1020.

Williams, J. I. (1981). Family medicine in Canada. *Marriage and Family Review, 4,* 163-187.

Wolfe, S., & Badgley, R. F. (1973). *The family doctor.* Toronto: Macmillan.

Wright, D. D., & Kane, R. L. (1982). Predicting outcome of primary care. *Medical Care, 20,* 180-187.

16 An Example of Assessing
     Health Care Delivery

ANTHONY J. REID

In Chapter 15, Dr. Williams reviewed studies of particular models and issues in primary health care delivery in the United States and Canada, looking specifically at the effects of large-scale interventions—such as the introduction of health care policy—on health care delivery. This chapter describes an example of assessment of an intervention in health care delivery in a primary care setting.

The role of family doctors in obstetrics has been declining, raising the need to evaluate the quality of care they provide. This chapter describes a study that addressed the question: "Do family physicians manage intrapartum care in women at low risk differently than do obstetricians and are there any differences in the outcomes?" (Reid, Carroll, Ruderman, & Murray, 1989).

The issues included the following: What is the appropriate study design to answer this question? What process measures should be used to assess the style of care? What final outcome measures would give an accurate picture of quality of care? How should both process measures and outcome measures be defined and recorded? What were the links between them?

Design

Our goal was to compare rates of interventions, and maternal and neonatal outcomes, between maternity cases handled either by family physicians or by obstetricians.

A randomized controlled trial would have been the strongest study design, but it was unlikely that patients would have allowed themselves to be assigned for their care, nor would ethics committees have approved such a course. Accordingly, a retrospective cohort design based on hospital records was chosen as the next strongest design, recognizing that we could not eliminate the bias created by maternity patients' choice in type of caregiver. For instance, it was felt that some women chose an obstetrician because of perceived greater competence, while others chose a family physician hoping to reduce unnecessary interventions. To counter this inherent problem, we tried to ensure that the two groups were equivalent in terms of medical and obstetric risk, the most important factors likely to affect outcomes. Also, this design does have an advantage in that the physicians involved did not know they were being studied, so that the "Hawthorne effect" was avoided.

SETTING

The study samples were drawn from three downtown Toronto hospitals where family physicians and obstetricians worked on the same labor floors with the same nursing staff. The physicians were a mixture of academic and community practitioners. These hospitals were chosen due to the range of services available, our access to records, and our experience working there. All three handled large numbers of deliveries, including low-risk births attended by obstetricians, so that a large sample size was readily obtainable.

While this setting may not reflect exact practice methods in other locales, many physicians are trained in such centers, and it was likely that it was reasonably representative of most Canadian hospitals.

SAMPLE

The sample of patients cared for by family physicians was taken from all women delivering at the three hospitals during a one-year period, while obstetricians' patients were selected by using random number tables to pick charts. For both groups, a woman had to be classified as "low risk" based on both her Ontario Antenatal Record and her history and physical at the time of being admitted in active labor. Only women in Category A (those with *no predictable risk*) were included. If there were any doubts, a patient was excluded. The selection process continued until there were an equal number of women in the two groups.

The questions arise: "Does this method identify all the women at any risk at the onset of labor?" "Were the groups comparable?" We feel that, by using both the antenatal form as well as the hospital-based documentation at the onset of labor, any women at risk in either group would have been noted.

The results appeared to confirm our impression of medical and obstetric equivalence, in that the proportions of women in each group were the same for gestational age at onset of labor, blood pressure at admission, and infant birth weights. The groups did differ, however, in some ways: The family physicians' group had more younger women, more primiparas, and a greater proportion of those of lower socioeconomic status (as determined by whether they were receiving social assistance or requested a ward versus a private room). All these factors would, if anything, tend to make the outcomes of the family physician cases worse.

An issue that was important for the whole study, as well as in risk identification, was the use of hospital records as a source of information. In the absence of a prospective design, it was impossible to standardize our data collection any more than was done in routine hospital practice; we had to rely on the accuracy of self-reported care by the physicians on the standard antenatal and labor and delivery forms. We noted, however, that nurses recorded much of the data on these forms; this should have improved the standardization of the data entry within each hospital. Also, much of the information was recorded on summary forms, which made documentation easier.

PROCESS MEASURES

Assessment of the type of care delivered was made through comparing frequencies of a number of interventions. These included artificial rupture of membranes, induction, augmentation, continuous electronic fetal monitoring (CEFM), low forceps, vacuum extraction, and episiotomy. These were chosen because they are commonly performed and their use has been the source of some controversy (e.g., episiotomy—Harrison, Brennan, North,

Table 16.1 Selected Outcomes

Intervention	Family Physician Group (n = 1115) Number (%)	Obstetrician (n = 1250) Number (%)	p
1. Low forceps or Vacuum Extractor (No rotations, mid-forceps)			
Primiparas	126 (21)	183 (31)	< 0.001
Multiparas	46 (9)	122 (19)	< 0.001
2. Episiotomy			
Primiparas	413 (69)	429 (72)	N.S.
Multiparas	202 (39)	370 (57)	< 0.001
3. Spontaneous vaginal delivery	760 (68)	689 (55)	< 0.001
4. Cesarean section	76 (6.8)	96 (7.7)	N.S.
5. Neonatal birth weight (gm) (+SD)	3445 (453.1)	3462 (457.4)	N.S.
6. Admission to special care baby unit	44 (3.9)	43 (3.4)	N.S.

Reed, & Wickman, 1984; Sleep, Grant, Garcia, Elbourne, Spencer, & Chalmers, 1984—and CEFM—Banta & Thacker, 1979). As well, they were all explicitly recorded on labor and delivery forms, making documentation easier. (See Table 16.1 for selected interventions.) Considerable effort was spent standardizing definitions and checking reliability for recording various interventions (and outcomes) to ensure consistently accurate recording.

OUTCOME MEASURES

Accurate assessment of the quality of maternity care is exceedingly difficult; there are many outcomes that give some indication of this but no gold standard that gives an accurate global rating (Patrick, 1988; Williams, 1991).

This study recorded three types of outcomes: (a) those describing the actual process (often linked to the intervention rates), such as length of second and third stages of labor, or rates of spontaneous vaginal delivery versus cesarean section; (b) those describing maternal events, such as perineal tear rates or postpartum hemorrhage; and (c) those related to the newborn, including birth weight and APGAR scores (see Table 16.1).

The most important outcome, we felt, was the rate of admission to the special care baby unit (SCBU), which has been used in previous studies and has been shown to be reproducible and reasonably sensitive (Klein, Lloyd, Redman, Bull, & Turnbull, 1983). We refined it further by checking the charts in each case and recording the indications for the admission for comparison. This was also done for intubation rates.

Unfortunately, especially in the area of neonatal outcomes, no one measure gives an accurate picture of quality of care during labor. APGARs are known to be inaccurate in predicting the long-term well-being of a baby (many babies who are "asphyxiated" at birth do well while others who are not develop neurological damage; Canadian Medical Protective Association and the American Academy for Cerebral Palsy and Developmental Medicine, 1988). As well, it was recognized that admission to the SCBU may be overly sensitive, with some babies not really needing it. It seemed, from our detailed follow-up, however, that the proportions of indications were very similar in each group, so there did not seem to be significant bias affecting either one. An ideal outcome would accurately reflect the quality of care during the labor and delivery process, with accurate prediction of long-term development in the child. Because no such measure exists, we had to be satisfied with the proxy measures described.

Because admission to SCBUs was felt to be the most sensitive marker for serious newborn outcomes, it was decided that this should be used for sample size calculation. We calculated that, for an outcome with a frequency of 5%, sample sizes of 1,200 per group would detect a 50% difference in rates for a p (α) of 0.05 and a power of 0.8. We felt that this was a reasonably small clinical difference; this was agreed to by our expert consultants (family physicians and obstetricians). We also recognized that, with many outcomes being recorded, some might have been different by chance alone.

Findings

The results confirmed earlier findings (Franks & Eisinger, 1987; Phillips, Rice, & Layton, 1978; Wanderer & Suyehire, 1980) that, for women at low risk, family physicians intervened less frequently and presided over more spontaneous vaginal deliveries, while maternal and newborn outcomes were no different than in cases managed by obstetricians.

We felt these conclusions were justified by the strength of the study design. While it was not randomized, there were good indications that the groups were similar for medical and obstetric risk. We felt confident that the recordings of process and outcome measurements were accurate and reliable, as far as hospital records would allow. Calculation of a reasonable sample size gave us confidence we were not making a type II error when no difference was found.

Although this study initially was focused on health care delivery by practitioners to individuals, its results also raised significant health policy and research questions. If there were no benefits shown for a more interventionist style of practice in low-risk maternity cases, was this practice justified? Should low-risk births be handled by specialists, given the limitations on health care resources? What levels of interventions are appropriate for low-risk births? This last question requires new research, because most investigations have been concerned with high-risk problems.

One additional point is that, when designing studies to assess health care delivery, one must be prepared to accept the limitations imposed by the subject matter and data available. By carefully addressing methodological issues and explaining the rationales for the choices made, one enables the reader to assess their validity. When done properly, such studies can provide useful information for health planners and physicians.

References

Banta, H., & Thacker, S. (1979). Policies toward medical technology: The case of electronic fetal monitoring. *American Journal of Public Health, 69*(9), 931-935.

Canadian Medical Protective Association and the American Academy for Cerebral Palsy and Developmental Medicine. (1988). *Perinatal asphyxia: Its role in develop-*

mental deficits in children (Proceedings of a symposium held in Toronto, Ontario, October 26, 1988). *Canadian Medical Association Journal* (Supplement, pp. 3-10).

Franks, P., & Eisinger, S. (1987). Adverse perinatal outcomes: Is physician specialty a risk factor? *Journal of Family Practice, 24,* 152-156.

Harrison, R., Brennan, M., North, P., Reed, J., & Wickham, E. (1984). Is routine episiotomy necessary? *British Medical Journal, 288,* 1971-1975.

Klein, M., Lloyd, I., Redman, C., Bull, M., & Turnbull, A. (1983). A comparison of low risk pregnant women booked for delivery in two systems of care: Shared care (consultant) and integrated general practice unit [in two parts]. *British Journal of Obstetrics and Gynaecology, 90,* 118-128.

Patrick, J. (1988). *Reproductive care: Towards the 1990's* (Second report of the advisory committee on reproductive care). Toronto: Ontario Ministry of Health.

Phillips, W., Rice, G., & Layton, R. (1978). Audit of obstetric care and outcome in family medicine, obstetrics and general practice. *Journal of Family Practice, 6,* 1209-1216.

Reid, A., Carroll, J., Ruderman, J., & Murray, M. (1989). Differences in intrapartum obstetric care provided to women at low risk by family physicians and obstetricians. *Canadian Medical Association Journal, 140,* 625-633.

Sleep, J., Grant, A., Garcia, J., Elbourne, D., Spencer, J., & Chalmers, I. (1984). West Berkshire perineal management trial. *British Medical Journal, 289,* 587-590.

Wanderer, M., & Suyehire, J. (1980). Obstetrical care in a prepaid cooperative: A comparison between family practice residents, family physicians and obstetricians. *Journal of Family Practice, 11,* 601-606.

Williams, J. (1991). Health services research. In H. Troidl, W. Spitzer, B. McPeek, D. S. Mulder, & M. F. McNeally (Eds.), *Principles and practice of research: Strategies for surgical investigators* (2nd ed.). New York: Springer-Verlag.

17 Analyzing Large Data Sets

CHARLYN BLACK
LESLIE L. ROOS
WALTER ROSSER
EARL V. DUNN

In its broadest sense, *assessment* refers to determination of the "importance, size, or value" of a particular subject of appraisal (*Webster's New Collegiate Dictionary*, Woolf, 1980). Tugwell, Bennett, Sackett, and Haynes (1985) developed a framework that outlines the many types of research activities required to assess clinical interventions. The cycle begins with identification of an intervention and estimation of its potential to reduce the "modifiable" burden of illness. It then moves to studies of *efficacy* (assessment of whether the intervention works under ideal circumstances), *effectiveness* (assessment of whether the intervention works when provided in a real-world practice setting), and *efficiency* (assessment of the relationship between costs and effects of the intervention). Once these issues have been studied, monitoring—assessment of the extent to which the intervention is applied in an efficacious, effective, and efficient manner in actual practice—becomes important. Finally, the success of the intervention in actually reducing the burden of illness must be assessed.

Assessment of interventions in primary care requires an even wider focus than the assessment of the clinical interventions outlined above. Other types of "interventions" have an impact on the quality, effectiveness, and efficiency of care. These include decisions made by providers to structure the delivery of care in a given manner: for example, explicit practice policies as to whether or not to provide services such as house calls or obstetric care, use of a computerized system to prompt physicians to provide preventive care (McDowell, Newell, & Rosser, 1989a, 1989b), or a change in the practice scheduling system to enhance continuity of care. Still another type of "intervention" affects the environment in which primary care is practiced. Examples here would be the introduction of alternative organizational mechanisms (e.g., health service organizations), changes in fee schedules (e.g., alteration in reimbursement for interventions such as Pap smears), or the introduction of a home care program.

The assessment of interventions in primary care therefore encompasses a wide spectrum of activities, settings, and interventions, all of which have implications for the quality and effectiveness of care delivered to patients. This wide range of activities demands a correspondingly wide range of research data and methods.

Until recently, most research in primary care has relied on "primary" data collection—the gathering of data expressly for the purpose of conducting a given research project. Ever more sophisticated computer technology, however, has led to the existence of computerized health care data sets of varying scope, quality, and complexity. Vital records, health insurance claims, and medical records are stored in retrievable computerized form and, as such, are potentially available for use by researchers.

Analysis of large sets of routinely collected data provides many advantages over primary data collection. These secondary sources provide data that, in addition to being inexpensive and readily available, are often of high quality in terms of reliability and validity. In addition, they assure large sample sizes and can provide many years of data to enhance long-term follow-up of individuals.

There are, however, many potential pitfalls in using secondary data sources. Their analysis differs from more traditional approaches because they were not designed, collected, or organized for the purpose of answering specific research questions.

This chapter defines large data sets, identifies different types and describes their relevance for primary care research, and considers some of the important issues involved in analyzing them.

Large Data Sets

Several assumptions are made here about large data sets. First, they comprise data in computer-readable format. Second, they consist of more than 10,000 observations—sufficiently large that the costs and intricacies of computer processing are a significant issue. Finally, they are assumed to have been designed primarily for purposes other than studying the research question of interest.

What would be the characteristics of an ideal large data set to assess interventions in primary care? First, each patient would be specified by a unique number or set of personal identifiers and adequately characterized in terms of age, sex, residence, socioeconomic status, and general health status. Second, each provider and practice site would also be specified by unique identifiers and characterized in terms of variables recognized as relevant in the delivery of primary care (e.g., for practitioners: family practice training, years in practice, participation in continuing medical education, payment mechanism; for practices: location, group versus solo, provision of after-hours care). Finally, a comprehensive set of information on each encounter would be collected, including the patient's stated reason for the encounter, diagnostic services performed, provider's assessment of the problem, therapeutic interventions, patient disposition, and other relevant variables.

In addition to these features, coverage of an entire population would permit assessment of interventions from an epidemiological perspective, to determine who receives given interventions and who does not. Information pertaining to use of health care services beyond the primary level of care (e.g., hospitalization) would be useful to assess the impact of primary care interventions on the need for other services. Finally, collection of data over time would provide the ability to construct detailed histories for individuals and to study the impact of interventions over different periods of time.

Medical insurance data sets and computerized clinical data sets are the two main types of large data sets useful for assessment of interventions in primary care. While designed primarily to provide information for management, they have considerable applicability for research. The two have certain similarities in structure in that both contain observations on encounters, patients, and sometimes on providers. They differ, however, in the range and comprehensiveness of variables captured, the numbers and types of observations, and the period of time that they cover. These differences have important implications for research.

MEDICAL INSURANCE DATA SETS

Medical insurance data files contain a vast array of demographic, diagnostic, and service data and constitute a population-based data source for many provinces in Canada. They usually contain (a) basic data on the individuals covered, in a population registry file; (b) basic data on providers eligible to provide care, in a physician file; and (c) encounter data for ambulatory, hospital, and nursing home care, in claims files. These data can often be further broadened through linkage to other data sets such as cancer registries, vital statistics, and prescription drug plan records. Their features are outlined in Table 17.1.

In Manitoba, considerable expertise has been gained in using medical insurance data to assess surgical interventions (Roos & Roos, 1989). More recently, work has focused on assessing interventions at the primary care level. Cohen, Roos, MacWilliam, and Wajda (1991) used data from the provincial health insurance files in Manitoba to describe appropriateness of patterns of cervical screening according to published guidelines. Current research is monitoring adverse events following immunization of children as well as studying health outcomes attributable to receipt of the influenza vaccine among the elderly. The Province of Saskatchewan collects data on prescription drugs as part of its insured pharmaceutical program; several studies of the effects of various drug interventions have been conducted there and in other settings (Ray & Griffin, 1989). Examples of assessment of clinical interventions using medical insurance data such as these, however, are relatively rare—generally, these data provide relatively limited information about specific interventions.

The great strength of medical insurance data sets, however, lies in their ability to provide a system- and populationwide perspective to data analysis, particularly when they include both unique individual identifiers and an enrollment file (Roos & Roos, 1989). Such data permit estimation of loss to follow-up, identification of incident cases, delineation of use patterns such as use of hospital

Table 17.1 Features of Different Types of Large Data Sets in Primary Care Research

Administrative Data Sets	Clinical Practice Data Sets		
	Minimum Data Set for Clinical Practice	Enhanced Research Data Set	Targeted Research Data Set
• Contain minimal information on entire set of patients, providers, and encounters in a defined region for insurance billing purposes	• Contain a basic set of items required in the medical record for adequate patient management	• Contain a more comprehensive set of items captured uniformly on every patient and encounter to expand research capability	• Contain minimum or enhanced research items for all patients and encounters
• Permit identification of complete use patterns for individuals, including those who do not use the system	• Ideally, should be standardized across practices—not yet developed for primary care	• Standardized across patients and encounters within the practice	• Supplemented by collection of additional data in specified situations to address specific research questions
• No data collection activity required	• Moderate data collection activity required	• Major data collection activity required	• Major data collection activity required
• Limited data for assessment of primary care interventions	• Adequate data for assessment of primary care interventions	• Rich data for assessment of primary care interventions	• Very rich data for assessment of specific primary care interventions
• Observational research designs only	• Observational as well as experimental research designs possible	• Observational as well as experimental research designs possible	• Observational as well as experimental research designs possible
• Good generalizability of results	• Problems with generalizability of results	• Problems with generalizability of results	• Problems with generalizability of results

care, measurement of long-term outcomes, and research on both efficacy and effectiveness. Furthermore, they permit more complete assessment of interventions at the provider or practice level and the health care system level than do data sets from clinical practice.

CLINICAL PRACTICE DATA SETS

With the advent of personal computer systems that handle billing functions and capture components of patients' medical records, large computerized clinical practice data sets are becoming available for research (Barnett, 1984; Barnett, Winickoff, Dorsey, Morgan, & Lurie, 1978; Elmslie & Rosser, 1986; Pryor et al., 1985; Rosser & Fluker, 1984). These data sets are usually collected within a practice setting and have as their primary objective the organization of data necessary to deliver optimal medical care. There are endless permutations on these data sets: They vary in terms of comprehensiveness of variables collected, coding schemes used to capture diagnostic and other data, and software used. From a research perspective, three subsets can be identified (Table 17.1).

The simplest—and most common—form is referred to here as a "minimum data set for clinical practice" and contains a basic set of items for patient management. Although these data sets have been used to provide useful information for research, they are limited by the lack of a standardized approach for data collection. Standardization would encourage collection of a more uniform and comprehensive set of variables and permit research using aggregations of data sets by different practices. The Health Care Financing Administration in the United States considers this a priority for primary care research and is in the process of developing a recommended Uniform Ambulatory Medical Care Minimum Data Set. The project will define a common core of those items most likely to be needed by a variety of users for multiple applications, with uniform definitions for inclusion in the records of all ambulatory health care.

A second level of clinical practice data set, an "enhanced research data set," involves collection of a more comprehensive set of variables on every patient and encounter. Its increased detail makes this type of data set more useful for research purposes. For instance, patients may be characterized more fully in terms of socioeconomic and general health status (Nelson et al., 1987), and additional variables relating to encounters may be captured, such as the patient's reason for the visit, intervention(s) provided (including diagnostic, therapeutic, and administrative services), and patient disposition. To this end, the World Organization of National Colleges, Academies and Academic Associations of General Practitioners/Family Physicians (WONCA) has done developmental work on a classification system for patient reason for encounter (which is not yet available) and another that records data about interventions and the "process" of care (WONCA, 1986). More accurate information regarding the provider's definition of the problem or diagnosis may be obtained by capturing multiple diagnoses (medical insurance data usually capture only a single diagnosis for ambulatory claims) and/or by capturing data in a format more appropriate to requirements in the ambulatory care setting (WONCA, 1983).

A third level of clinical practice data set, a "targeted research data set," takes advantage of the ability of computerized systems to identify specific patients, medical problems, or interventions for collection of more specialized data. For instance, in a study on treatment of hypertension within a practice, the computer may identify individuals who (a) have diastolic blood pressures falling within a certain range, (b) are in a defined age group, and (c) are receiving a specific intervention. In addition to routine data, more detailed information may be collected for specific situations of interest to the researcher, by using either a patient survey or a customized encounter sheet that collects information from the provider. In this manner, the researcher gains considerable control over the collection of data and can link primary data collection to routinely collected data. This approach also supports research designs that rely on random allocation of interventions and prospective data collection, thereby permitting more rigorous assessment of primary care interventions.

The limitation of all clinical practice data sets is that they only provide information for the set of encounters in a particular practice; they do not capture contacts that patients may have at other practice sites, and they are unlikely to capture use of other health services, which are important potential confounders in studying primary care interventions. This leads to problems in identifying the denominators of primary care practices and in determining the generalizability of findings. Furthermore, findings are less generalizable than those derived from systemwide administrative data. They may be generalized only to similar practice settings, not to other practice settings and population groups.

The strengths of medical insurance and clinical practice data sets are therefore complementary. While the former offer system- and populationwide coverage, they contain only limited data to assess interventions in primary care. The latter, on the other hand, offer rich and detailed information to characterize the patient, the encounter, and the intervention but are limited in their scope and generalizability. Future research endeavors are likely to benefit from these complementary features by linking these two types of data. For example, research on the appropriateness of patterns of cervical screening yields a different perspective when studied using a clinical practice data base (which captures only a subset of encounters for a given patient) than when studied using an administrative data base that captures the total set of encounters for a given patient (Cohen et al., 1991). Both perspectives are relevant and bring useful information to the analysis.

Issues to Be Considered

The term *analysis* has been used in this discussion to refer to a large and complex set of research activities that must be executed with great caution when applied to secondary data sets. The same vigilance that goes into planning research based on primary data collection must be exercised when planning research that relies on analysis of existing administrative or clinical practice data.

Discussion of all of the issues involved is beyond the scope of this chapter; they include attention to data quality, research design, control of differences in case mix and severity, statistical and analytic issues as well as approaches to data management. Most of these have been previously well described (Connell, Diehr, & Hart, 1987; Feinstein, 1989; Institute of Medicine, 1985; Roos & Roos, 1989). This discussion will focus on issues that are more specific to the analysis of primary care data sets.

DATA QUALITY

Data quality is an issue for both medical insurance and clinical practice data sets and must always be assessed. Because information is more likely to be recorded accurately if it is used, variables that are meaningful to clinical practice are also likely to be reliable and valid for research purposes. Collection of additional variables that are useful for research but not used by clinicians should therefore be kept to a minimum.

The accuracy of diagnostic information depends on both the physicians who produce it and the clerks who record it. In insurance data sets, diagnoses on ambulatory claims are likely to be less accurate than diagnoses on hospital records. Because of this, ambulatory diagnoses are useful but at a much more generalized level. Several diagnostic grouping systems for ambulatory data have been developed to make ICD-9 coding of diagnoses more useful for primary care. Schneeweis, Rosenblatt, Cherkin, Kirkwood, and Hart (1983) have developed a system to cluster ICD-9 diagnoses into clinically meaningful diagnostic groups. This system has been claimed to reduce spurious variation resulting from idiosyncratic diagnostic labeling habits of providers. As an alternative, use of the International Classification of Health Problems in Primary Care (WONCA, 1983) to capture diagnostic data in primary care may address validity problems that abound with ICD-9 coding.

DELINEATING EPISODES OF CARE

Many investigators of use and quality of medical care advocate the use of "episodes of care" in the analysis of ambulatory utilization data, especially to study interventions for specific health problems. An *episode* may be defined as a set of medical services received continuously by a patient in response to a particular request (Stoddart, 1975) or as "a block of one or more medical services received by an individual during a period of relatively continuous contact with one or more providers of service, in relation to a particular medical problem or condition" (Solon, Feeney, Jones, Rigg, & Sheps, 1967). Therefore, it differs from an episode of illness, which is patient defined. The use history of an individual may be regarded as being composed of discrete episodes of care provided for one or more medical problems, conditions, requests, or episodes of illness.

Approaches to the creation of episodes of care have varied, depending on the data sources used and the information available. They usually involve development of algorithms that consider diagnostic and temporal information for grouping visits into logical episodes. From a clinical perspective, however, many of the methods available appear to be overly simplistic and do not adequately handle either chronic conditions or patients who have multiple problems.

CONTROLLING FOR DIFFERENCES IN CASE MIX AND SEVERITY

Controlling for possible differences in patient characteristics is critical when comparing primary care interventions in different practices. Although ambulatory insurance data provide very limited information to make these adjustments, measures of comorbidity and severity have been shown to compare favorably with those relying on primary data collection (Roos, Sharp, Cohen, & Wajda, 1989). Most of the measures developed to date, however, require hospital data and are therefore not useful for characterizing ambulatory populations. More recently, a case-mix measure has been developed that uses data from ambulatory encounters. It requires information on a patient's age, sex, and ambulatory diagnoses over a defined period of time, all of which may be obtained from administrative data sets (Starfield, Weiner, Mumford, & Steinwachs, 1991; Weiner, Starfield, Steinwachs, & Mumford, 1991). This measure holds promise to control for case mix using data sets that contain limited information on each patient and encounter.

The availability of more specific variables in clinical practice data sets provides increased ability to control for case mix and severity. Although standard measures have not been agreed upon, considerable work has gone into testing items in clinical practice settings (Horn, Buckle, & Carver, 1988; Nelson et al., 1987; Parkerson et al., 1989; Stewart et al., 1989). Further refinement of these measures is necessary because of the importance of having reliable and valid measures to control for the burden of illness in a practice population. Most of these indices require the collection of additional variables, which has implications for the cost and quality of data systems.

ETHICAL CONSIDERATIONS

With the development of computerized clinical data sets, the boundary between patient care and research becomes blurred. Special consideration must be given to assure the ethical conduct of research and to protect the confidentiality of individuals on whom the data are collected. With research using insurance data sets, all requests for data must be approved both by an ethics committee and a committee that monitors access to the data; the data are provided with elimination and/or scrambling of patient and provider identifiers; and special precautions are taken to safeguard the data in terms of physical security and limitations on access. Research that uses clinical practice data sets must respect the boundary between research and clinical activities by using approaches parallel to those outlined above. Quick "analysis" of clinical data sets is likely to violate ethical codes and the patient's right to confidentiality.

Summary and Conclusions

Assessment of interventions in primary care involves a broad range of research questions, ranging from defining the level of need for the intervention, to determining its effectiveness, and to monitoring its application in practice. In addition to interventions at the clinical level, interventions at the level of the provider, the practice, or the health care system affect primary care and patient outcomes. The data requirements to assess interventions are therefore substantial.

Large computerized health care data sets containing information that is routinely collected in medical insurance agencies and clinical practices are becoming increasingly available to researchers to meet these needs for data. Their maintenance, analysis, and improvement represent an inexpensive and useful way to enhance and promote assessment of interventions, and research using them is likely to generate important new knowledge for primary care.

References

Barnett, G. O. (1984). The application of computer-based medical-record systems in ambulatory practice. *New England Journal of Medicine, 310*, 1643-1650.

Barnett, G. O., Winickoff, R. N., Dorsey, J. L., Morgan, M. M., & Lurie, R. S. (1978). Quality assurance through automated monitoring and concurrent feedback using a computer-based medical information system. *Medical Care, 16*, 962-970.

Cohen, M., Roos, N. P., MacWilliam, L., & Wajda, A. (1991). *Assessing the appropriateness of physicians' practice patterns for Pap testing.* Unpublished manuscript.

Connell, F. A., Diehr, P., & Hart, L. G. (1987). The use of large data bases in health care studies. *Annual Review of Public Health, 8*, 51-74.

Elmslie, T., & Rosser, W. W. (1986). Computerization of family practice. *Canadian Medical Association Journal, 134*, 221-224.

Feinstein, A. R. (1989). Para-analysis, faute de mieux, and the perils of riding on a data barge. *Journal of Clinical Epidemiology, 42*, 10.

Horn, S. D., Buckle, J. M., & Carver, C. M. (1988). Ambulatory severity index: Development of an ambulatory case mix system. *Journal of Ambulatory Care Management, 11*, 53-62.

Institute of Medicine. (1985). *Assessing medical technologies.* Washington, DC: National Academy Press.

McDowell, I., Newell, C., & Rosser, W. (1989a). Computerized reminders to encourage cervical screening in family practice. *Journal of Family Practice, 28*, 420-424.

McDowell, I., Newell, C., & Rosser, W. (1989b). A randomized trial of computerized reminders for blood pressure screening in primary care. *Medical Care, 27*, 297-305.

Nelson, E., Wasson, J., Keller, A., Clark, D., Dietrich, A., Stewart, A., & Zubkoff, M. (1987). Assessment of function in routine clinical practice: Description of the COOP chart method and preliminary findings. *Journal of Chronic Diseases, 40*(1), 55S-63S.

Parkerson, G. R., Jr., Michener, J. L., Wu, L. R., Finch, J. N., Muhlbaier, L. H., Magruder-Habib, K., Kertesz, J. W., Clapp-Channing, N., Morrow, D. S., Chen, A. L. T., & Jokerst, E. (1989). Associations among family support, family stress, and personal functional health status. *Journal of Clinical Epidemiology, 42*, 217-229.

Pryor, D. P., Califf, R. M., Harrell, F. E., Hlatky, M. A., Lee, K. L., Mark, D. B., & Rosati, R. A. (1985). Clinical data bases: Accomplishments and unrealized potential. *Medical Care, 23*, 623-647.

Ray, W. A., & Griffin, M. R. (1989). Use of Medicaid data for pharmoco-epidemiology. *American Journal of Epidemiology, 129*, 837-849.

Roos, L. L., & Roos, N. P. (1989). Large data bases and research on surgery. In I. M. Rutkow (Ed.), *Socioeconomics of surgery.* St. Louis, MO: Mosby.

Roos, L. L., Sharp, S. M., Cohen, M. M., & Wajda, A. (1989). Risk adjustment in claims-based research: The search for efficient approaches. *Journal of Clinical Epidemiology, 42*, 1193-1206.

Rosser, W. W., & Fluker, G. (1984). Software for family practice: A decade of development. *Canadian Family Physician, 30*, 2567-2571.

Schneeweis, R., Rosenblatt, R. A., Cherkin, D. C., Kirkwood, C. R., & Hart, G. (1983). Diagnosis clusters: A new tool for analyzing the content of ambulatory medical care. *Medical Care, 21*, 105-122.

Solon, J. A., Feeney, J. J., Jones, S. H., Rigg, R. D., & Sheps, C. G. (1967). Delineating episodes of medical care. *American Journal of Public Health, 57,* 401-408.

Starfield, B., Weiner, J., Mumford, L., & Steinwachs, D. (1991). Ambulatory care groups: A categorization of diagnoses for research and management. *Health Service Research, 26,* 53-74.

Stewart, A. L., Greenfield, S., Hays, R. D., Wells, K., Rogers, W. H., Berry, S., McGlynn, E. A., & Ware, J. E. (1989). Functional status and well-being of patients with chronic conditions. *Journal of the American Medical Association, 262,* 907-913.

Stoddart, G. L. (1975). *An episodic approach to the demand for medical care.* Unpublished doctoral thesis, University of British Columbia.

Tugwell, P., Bennett, K. J., Sackett, D. L., & Haynes, R. B. (1985). The measurement iterative loop: A framework for the critical appraisal of need, benefits, and costs of health interventions. *Journal of Chronic Diseases, 38,* 4.

Weiner, J. P., Starfield, B. H., Steinwachs, D. M., & Mumford, L. M. (1991). Development and application of a population-oriented measure of ambulatory care case-mix. *Medical Care, 29,* 452-472.

Woolf, H. B. (Ed.). (1980). *Webster's new collegiate dictionary.* Springfield, MA: G & C Merriam.

World Organization of National Colleges, Academies and Academic Associations of General Practitioners/Family Physicians (WONCA), in collaboration with the World Health Organization (WHO). (1983). *ICHPPC-2-Defined.* Oxford: Oxford University Press.

World Organization of National Colleges, Academies and Academic Associations of General Practitioners/Family Physicians (WONCA), in collaboration with the North American Primary Care Research Group (NAPCRG). (1986). *IC-Process-PC.* Oxford: Oxford University Press.

18 The Sioux Lookout Project as an Example of a Large Data Set

EARL V. DUNN

Chapter 17 discussed theoretical aspects of several types of large data sets, their interrelation, and some of the problems associated with them. This chapter describes an actual example of a large data set and examines how such information can be used. The data set in question was derived from nearly 150,000 encounters with the health system during a 3-year period for a population of more than 12,000 people living in an isolated area of Canada. Its purpose was to analyze the effects of a "telemedicine" communication system introduced into the area in 1978.

The Setting

The Sioux Lookout Zone in northwestern Ontario covers an area of 385,000 square kilometers, almost as large as California. The region is a subarctic boreal forest, dotted with numerous lakes and rivers, and has temperatures that reach –40°C in winter. It is sparsely populated, with only 12,000 people, mostly native Canadians. Its hub is the town of Sioux Lookout with a population of about 4,000; another 27 communities lie from 31 to more than 750 kilometers to the north, with most being more than 200 kilometers from the town. Transportation is difficult, as few of the communities are connected by roads. The larger ones at least have dry land airstrips, but the smaller ones are served only by planes with floats or skis.

The medical center serving the area is the 50-bed Sioux Lookout Zone hospital. (The nearest tertiary care hospital is in Winnipeg, 320 kilometers away.) The 27 northern communities have no doctors in residence; doctors visit the larger ones several times a month and the smaller ones on a less frequent basis. In 1980, seven of the larger communities had nursing stations with from two to five nurses, while the others had indigenous, minimally trained health aides providing daily care.

There are more than 50,000 encounters with the health system in a year in the Sioux Lookout Zone. Patients are usually seen initially in their own communities, then transferred to the zone hospital if necessary. In the case of maternal care, prenatal care is provided locally and then the mother is transferred to the zone hospital for delivery.

The Intervention

Between 1978 and 1980, a research project was set up to study the effects of telecommunication technology in health care. As part of this project, a slow-scan video system was installed in several of the Sioux Lookout Zone communities. Slow-scan video is a technology whereby a video picture—such as views of X-rays, EKGs, or skin rashes—can be transmitted via telephone lines. The system was installed in three of the seven northern nursing stations, in the zone hospital, and in an adult and a pediatric hospital in Toronto, 1,500 kilometers distant. Medical consultations, educational rounds, and social programs were conducted using this system during the 3-year research period.

The purpose of the Telemedicine Project was to describe the usage of this technology and to conduct a costs/effects study comparing the three communities whose nursing stations were set up with it against the four that were not. Comparisons included costs, X-rays taken, patient transfers, type of transfer, and length of stay in hospital.

Data Collection

The data collection book for the project was set up based on an existing daybook with additions for the extra information needed. The data included visits to all health workers (doctors, nurses, and health aides) in all communities and recorded all diagnoses, managements, communications, referrals, and transfers. Two copies were made; one was retained at the health facility and the other sent for data input and analysis. The diagnoses and managements were coded by one person, and an extensive error-checking routine was established. In addition, data were available on all admissions to the zone hospital.

Examples of Analyses

This chapter does not include detailed discussion of the findings of the Telemedicine Project: interested readers are referred to Conrath, Dunn, and Higgins (1983), Dunn, Acton, Conrath, Higgins, and Bain (1980), and Dunn, Conrath, Acton, Higgins, and Bain (1980), and Higgins (1980). Rather, it presents examples to illustrate the principles outlined by Drs. Black, Roos, Rosser, and Dunn in Chapter 17. All these examples are uses of the data from the basic data collection forms alone.

MINIMAL DATA SET

The records of patient identification, diagnoses, and services provided constituted the "minimal data set" as outlined by Dr. Black et al. Table 18.1 shows an example. These data, which were produced as a monthly report for the zone hospital administration and the nurses, were used for planning and for deciding on priorities for educational programs. Each nursing station received these reports for its own community to assist in its planning.

FULL CLINICAL DATA

The full clinical data set was used in several ways. Some of the data were incorporated into the monthly reports. Information on

Table 18.1 Diagnoses by ICHPPC Class: Frequency and Percentage

Class	Nurse Number (%)	Health Aide Number (%)	Doctor Number (%)	Total Number (%)
1 Infective	12,180 (12.4)*	3,042 (11.5)	1,263 (8.5)	15,598 (11.2)
2 Neoplasms	744 (0.7)	8 (0.0)	214 (1.4)	965 (0.7)
3 Endocrine	2,829 (2.9)	354 (1.3)	729 (4.9)	3,889 (2.8)
4 Blood	1,346 (1.4)	98 (0.4)	206 (1.4)	1,650 (1.2)
5 Mental	2,468 (2.5)	373 (1.4)	369 (2.5)	3,198 (2.3)
6 Nervous	13,483 (13.7)	2,039 (7.7)	2,616 (17.5)	18,138 (13.0)
7 Circulatory	6,694 (6.8)	1,101 (4.2)	1,663 (11.1)	9,458 (6.8)
8 Respiratory	20,672 (21.0)	6,487 (24.6)	2,122 (14.2)	25,037 (21.0)
9 Digestive	5,228 (5.3)	1,277 (4.8)	728 (4.9)	7,233 (5.2)
10 Urinary	12,731 (12.9)	1,855 (7.0)	2,593 (17.4)	17,129 (12.3)
11 Pregnancy	4,511 (4.6)	288 (1.1)	962 (6.4)	5,757 (4.1)
12 Skin	10,049 (10.2)	2,902 (11.0)	1,236 (8.3)	14,187 (10.2)
13 Musculoskeletal	5,298 (5.4)	1,251 (4.7)	1,212 (8.1)	7,761 (5.6)
14 Congenital	421 (0.4)	8 (0.0)	314 (2.1)	743 (0.5)
15 Perinatal	99 (0.1)	9 (0.0)	18 (0.1)	127 (0.1)
16 Signs and symptoms	19,800 (20.1)	10,363 (39.3)	3,378 (22.6)	33,541 (24.0)
17 Accidents	12,292 (12.5)	2,284 (8.7)	1,140 (7.6)	15,716 (11.3)
18 Supplementary	29,554 (30.0)	4,745 (18.0)	4,692 (31.4)	38,991 (27.9)
Total diagnoses	127,573	33,313	19,268	180,163
Patients seen	98,338 (70.4)	26,345 (18.9)	14,935 (10.7)	139,618

*Percentage of diagnoses per patient seen by provider class; the column percentages total to more than 100% because, in the ICHPPC classification, a number of diagnoses (e.g., warts, prenatal care) appear in more than one class.

the diagnoses and management was used in the planning of educational programs and in assisting different health workers in management practices. For example, the minimally trained health aides would often diagnose symptoms. Fever was their most common diagnosis, especially for patients who were referred and transferred. In fact, for patients transferred by health aides, 7 of the 10 most common diagnostic labels were symptoms. Educational programs and clinical algorithms were devised to assist these workers to deal with symptoms and to increase their diagnostic skills.

More sophisticated analyses were done to compare the quality of care provided by the various types of health workers. Using trajectory analysis to follow patients over time (Higgins, 1980), we

Table 18.2 Treatment for Upper Respiratory Infection

	Antibiotics Given on First Visit	Number of Episodes Number (%)	Subsequent Diagnosis of Bronchitis or Pneumonia During Episode Number (%)
Nurse	No	3,339 (84)	303 (9) $p = .04$
	Yes	614 (16)	64 (10) $p = > .10$
Health Aide	No	1,504 (85)	109 (7)
	Yes	263 (15)	28 (10)

analyzed outcomes for several diagnoses including upper respiratory infections and lacerations. For the former, we ascertained the number of patients who developed pneumonia during the same episode of care, and, for the latter, the number who developed subsequent infections, then compared the different levels of provider to see if there were important areas of differing outcomes (Dunn & Higgins, 1986, 1987).

Table 18.2 shows that, for upper respiratory infections, nurses and health aides had similar use of antibiotics as part of management, and the number of patients who were seen and had a diagnosis of pneumonia were similar. Thus we concluded that, for this diagnosis, the minimally trained health aides were providing care of as good quality as the nurses—the system of supervision and monitoring of care seemed to be working. The results for lacerations gave similar results.

SPECIALIZED DATA FIELDS

The data related to the use and evaluation of the slow-scan system were considered in several ways. The major study involved the cost implications. Tables 18.3 and 18.4 display the results of a comparison for those communities with or without the new technology on the use of X-rays and transfers of patients, respectively. Table 18.3 supported our hypothesis that the number of X-rays taken would increase in those nursing stations with the technology. What we had not predicted was that the number of patients transferred following an X-ray would also increase in these same

Table 18.3 Percentage of Patients Given X-Rays

	1978	1979	1980	1980–1978	Rank
Communities With Slow-Scan:					
New Osnaburgh	5.551	5.601	4.713	−0.838	3
Big Trout Lake	6.260	5.632	6.689	0.429	2
Sandy Lake	3.016	4.321	4.531	1.515	1
Communities Without Slow-Scan:					
Round Lake	4.176	3.099	2.321	−1.855	5
Pikangikum	6.333	5.951	3.866	−2.467	7
Fort Hope	4.883	3.835	2.875	−2.008	6
Lansdowne House	3.207	5.293	1.850	−1.357	4

NOTE: $P[WRST] < 6 = .0286$.

communities, as indicated by Table 18.4. Similar analyses were completed for eight other specific hypotheses. In addition, studies were completed that looked at the costs of the equipment and its operation, routine care, nursing station admissions, and hospitalizations. The results showed that there were no cost savings with this equipment but that benefits in education and socialization related to it were obtained without overall increase in costs. An indication of the success of this experimental system is that, 10 years later, without extra funds, the Telemedicine Project continues.

LINKAGES TO OTHER DATA SETS

In their chapter, Drs. Black, Roos, Rosser, and Dunn pointed out that the benefits of analyzing large data sets can be enhanced considerably if the data can be linked to other data sets for further analysis. In the Sioux Lookout Telemedicine Project, by using a unique patient identifier, we could link the data from the remote communities to the administrative, transport, and hospitalization data, thereby making comparisons possible between several different data sets. For example, one study looked at the association between a mother's absence from the community for perinatal care and the health of her children left behind in the community (Higgins, Dunn, & Conrath, 1981).

Table 18.4 Percentage of Patients Transferred Following X-Rays

	1978	1979	1980	1980-1978	Rank
Communities With Slow-Scan:					
New Osnaburgh	1.575	7.971	5.426	3.851	7
Big Trout Lake	5.316	5.138	6.954	1.638	6
Sandy Lake	3.830	5.696	4.192	0.362	4
Communities Without Slow-Scan:					
Round Lake	14.365	4.000	14.000	–0.365	2
Pikangikum	2.979	2.146	3.650	0.671	5
Fort Hope	1.905	4.225	1.802	–0.103	3
Lansdowne House	9.302	10.667	0.000	–9.302	1

NOTE: P[WRST]<17 = .9714.

In another large study, the clinical data set was used with several other data sources to develop an explanatory model for health status in the community using the encounter data as one measure of illness behavior (Duxbury, 1983). As might be expected, this study indicated that the health care system itself had less effect on illness in the community than did other factors such as housing and nutrition. It is surprising that the factors of isolation and paradoxically of having a community center and/or a radio station were more closely associated with good health than were the number of health care workers or other direct measures of health system availability and accessibility.

Problems

Whenever a large data set is being accumulated and analyzed, problems are inevitable, and care must be taken to minimize their number and consequences. These problems include incomplete data, errors, and problems with analysis.

A relatively complete data set is essential so that the analyses can be trusted. When dealing with a large data set, extra precautions must be taken because large numbers can more easily obscure and hide missing or incomplete data in individual cases. To minimize this problem, we took several measures. As mentioned, the main data collection instrument was based on the previously used daybook and was changed as little as possible; in fact, it was organized so that, even with the additional data required for the Telemedicine Project, it took less time than before for the nurses to complete. Before, the nurses had spent several hours a day per community preparing reports for the zone administration; now, if they provided us with complete data, we could produce those reports by computer, which gave them an incentive to fill in the forms as completely as possible. The monthly reports that were produced were not only useful to the nurses, they also allowed for small subsets of data to be considered and thus for missing data to be noted. Data were cross-checked with other similar-sized communities, and historical data for the same community were analyzed for obvious, sudden changes. Every opportunity was taken to remind the nurses and other health workers of the need for maintaining accurate and complete entries.

Compared with missing data, errors in data are insidious and difficult to spot and to correct; thus several strategies were used to identify them. The customary method of examination of outliers was used, with limits placed on all diagnoses and managements whenever feasible. For example, sex limits were placed on all sex-related diseases, and age or sex limits placed on medications, such as a limit of females for certain hormones, and an age limit of more than 20 years for digoxin. Each month, the age and sex limits were run against all new data, and those records with data outside the limits were manually compared with the original records. If coding or keypunching errors were identified, they were corrected; if there were no such errors, the record was checked at the source. Halfway through the project, a random selection of more than 1,000 records were checked and found to have an error rate of less than 1%.

The procedures and methods of data analysis in large data sets are problematic, both because of the difficulties of manipulating the data and because of the computer requirements. The latter is becoming less of an issue but is still relevant. In our case, we had major problems because, in the early 1980s, computer memory and speeds were not what they are today. For a major data run for all 150,000 records, we required a university mainframe and took up most of its capacity for several hours. We were allowed to run a full program only during the early morning hours, and, if something went wrong or the program needed changing, we often had to wait several days before we could run it again, which made extensive data analysis very time-consuming. This is still a problem that must be dealt with when considering large data sets.

Conclusion

Computerization has made it much easier to collect, organize, and analyze data collections of many records. As more of these are accumulated, it becomes essential that researchers know how to use them to achieve the desired information. We are still in the early stages of understanding in this area, and much work needs to be done. It is hoped that this chapter and the previous one can be a useful starting point for those setting out to perform such studies.

References

Conrath, D. W., Dunn, E. V., & Higgins, C. (1983). *Evaluating telecommunications technology in medicine.* Dedham, MA: Artech House.

Dunn, E. V., Acton, H., Conrath, D., Higgins, C., & Bain, H. (1980). The use of slow-scan video for CME in a remote area. *Journal of Medical Education, 55,* 493-495.

Dunn, E. V., Conrath, D. W., Acton, H., Higgins, C., & Bain, H. (1980). Telemedicine links patients in Sioux Lookout with doctors in Toronto. *Canadian Medical Association Journal, 122,* 484-486.

Dunn, E. V., & Higgins, C. A. (1986). Health problems encountered by three levels of providers in a remote setting. *American Journal of Public Health, 76,* 154-159.

Dunn, E. V., & Higgins, C. A. (1987). Comparisons of two types of nonphysician providers using episode based data. *Journal of Rural Health, 3,* 11-22.

Duxbury, L. (1983). *The relative effects of community characteristics and health care environment on Indian health and use of health care facilities in the Sioux Lookout Zone.* Unpublished doctoral thesis, University of Waterloo, Waterloo, Ontario.

Higgins, C. A. (1980). *Analysis of a remote health care system with telemedicine.* Unpublished doctoral thesis, University of Waterloo, Waterloo, Ontario.

Higgins, C., Dunn, E. V., & Conrath, D. W. (1981). Mother-child separation: A study in a remote health care setting. *Canadian Medical Association Journal, 125,* 1114-1117.

19 Meta-Analysis in Primary Care: Theory and Practice

ANDREW D. OXMAN
SYLVIE J. STACHENKO

Meta-analysis refers to the application of quantitative methods in summarizing research findings (Glass, 1976). It is not a specific technique but "a perspective that uses many techniques of measurement and statistical analysis" (Glass, McGaw, & Smith, 1981). The term was first suggested by Glass in 1976. Other terms used synonymously with *meta-analysis* include *pooling, overview,* and *quantitative synthesis.* There has been considerable debate as to which is preferable (Yusuf, Simon, & Ellenberg, 1987). Some investigators have expressed discomfort with the term, calling it a "junk word" and "etymological nonsense" (Nelder, 1988). Whatever its shortcomings, however, it is now in common use in the medical literature (Dickerson, Higgins, & Meinert, 1990), and in 1989 the U.S. National Library of Medicine introduced it as a MeSH indexing term (National Library of Medicine, 1989).

Meta-analytic approaches to summarizing research have generated considerable interest in the medical literature (L'Abbe, Detsky, & O'Rourke, 1987; Sacks, Berrier, Reitman, Ancona-Berk, & Chalmers, 1987; Thacker, 1988; Yusuf et al., 1987). Perhaps more important, there is a growing recognition that the same scientific principles apply both to meta-analyses and to traditional (narrative) literature reviews (Jackson, 1980; Mulrow, 1987; Oxman, 1989; Oxman & Guyatt, 1988). A literature review is a survey of research and follows the same principles that apply to an epidemiological survey in that a question must be clearly specified, a target population of information sources identified and accessed, appropriate information obtained from that population in an unbiased fashion, and conclusions derived. In meta-analyses, formal statistical analysis is used to help formulate conclusions.

As with any research study, there are a number of methodological decisions that must be made when undertaking a meta-analysis, and there are potential threats to validity associated with each decision (Cooper, 1989). This chapter will highlight the major issues and decisions to be made when undertaking a meta-analysis, illustrating them with examples from recently published literature, and will offer some pragmatic advice.

Protocol Development

Carrying out a meta-analysis involves a number of steps. As in any scientific endeavor, the methods to be used should be established beforehand.

An outline for a complete protocol for an overview is shown in Table 19.1. The first item is a review of prior reviews, which should inform the development of the overview and establish the rationale for undertaking it. This is analogous to reviewing previous research before preparing a protocol for "primary" research (research in which original data are collected and analyzed).

Because meta-analyses are retrospective analyses of data that have already been collected by others, it is important to make the process as rigorous and well defined as possible (Sacks et al., 1987). It is also necessary, however, to maintain a practical perspective. For each task in the protocol, the expenditure of resources that is required must be balanced against the magnitude of the associated threat to the overview's validity.

While every effort should be made to adhere to a predetermined protocol, it should be recognized that this will not always be possible or appropriate. Just as protocols for primary research must frequently be changed to adapt to unanticipated circumstances (such as problems with patient recruitment, data collection, or unexpected event rates), changes in an overview protocol must sometimes be made. Such changes should not be made on the basis of the results, however. Post hoc decisions (such as excluding

Table 19.1 Outline for an Overview Protocol

---

1. Objectives
2. Current state of knowledge
3. Study design
    3.1. General approach
    3.2. Study identification
    3.3. Study selection
    3.4. Study validation
    3.5. Data collection
    3.6. Analysis
    3.7. Inferences and presentation of results
4. Time chart for major activities
5. Budget

---

selected studies) that are made after their impact on the results is known are highly susceptible to bias and should be avoided. As a rule, all changes in the protocol should be documented and reported, and sensitivity analyses (L'Abbe et al., 1987) of the impact of such decisions on the results of the meta-analysis should be conducted when possible. *Sensitivity analysis* refers to the process of testing how sensitive the results of the meta-analysis are to changes in the way that the meta-analysis was done. Because there are bound to be differing opinions on the best approach to a particular meta-analysis, reviewers should always examine how robust their results are relative to key methodological decisions, such as including only randomized trials instead of both randomized and nonrandomized studies.

Identifying Studies

It is surprisingly difficult to locate all the published research in a particular area, even when the area is relatively circumscribed (such as all randomized control trials concerning a given therapy; Bernstein, 1988; De Neef, 1988; Dickerson, Hewitt, Mutch, Chalmers, & Chalmers, 1985; Kirpalani, Schmidt, McKibbon, Haynes, & Sinclair, 1989; Poynard & Conn, 1985). While an overview should include as many of the relevant primary studies as possible, it must be remembered that the more comprehensive a search strategy is, the less efficient it will be. Practically speaking, it is not possible to know when "100%" of the relevant studies for a particular topic have been located.

For most overviews, a variety of search strategies will be required. A reviewer normally will have accumulated a "file drawer" of relevant articles before undertaking a meta-analysis and should begin by noting text words that regularly appear in their titles and abstracts. These text words, and the key words with which the papers are indexed, can then be used to conduct a comprehensive MEDLINE search of the medical literature from 1966 to the current time. If appropriate, the same strategy can be used with other computerized data bases such as EMBASE (*Excerpta Medica* on-line). An excellent source to locate and determine the relevance of additional data bases is *Online Databases in the Medical and Life Sciences*, a directory of 795 data bases.

The reference lists of all articles obtained should be reviewed and additional relevant articles identified and retrieved. Frequently cited articles can be identified and *Index Medicus* can be used to search manually for articles published prior to 1966; and manual searches of key journals in which relevant research is likely to have been published can be used to ensure the comprehensiveness of the search. Studies such as theses, dissertations, and contract research studies should also be considered for inclusion.

One way to locate unpublished research is to construct a comprehensive list of relevant articles and send it with a letter to the first author of each paper, asking whether he or she knows of any work relevant to the area not included on the list. Other strategies include the use of relevant computerized data bases of unpublished studies, such as the U.S. National Cancer Institute's Physicians' Data Query Protocol Database, and writing or calling relevant professional and scientific organizations.

Two potential sources of bias to be aware of when searching for relevant studies are publication bias and selection bias. Unpublished studies may be systematically different than those appearing in peer-reviewed journals, not because their methodology was inferior but because their results were "negative." Research suggests that, of two studies that use the same methods to investigate a question, the one that yields "positive results" (refuting the null hypothesis) is more likely to be published and cited (Begg & Berlin, 1989; Dickerson, Chan, Chalmers, Sacks, & Smith, 1987; Easterbrook, Berlin, Gopalan, & Matthews, 1991). It thus behooves a reviewer to attempt to determine the extent of "publication bias" in the area of interest. Written reports of unpublished studies should be obtained if possible and their quality evaluated using the same criteria that are used to evaluate published research. Sensitivity analyses can be used to determine the impact of unpublished research on the overall results.

Selection bias refers to the finding that reviewers have a tendency to selectively cite references that support their own conclusions (Gotszche, 1987). To protect against this, titles of the reference lists obtained should, as a rule, be reviewed by two observers to ensure the reproducibility of the decisions that are made. Any article that either observer feels may be relevant should be retrieved.

The extent to which extensive searches for both published and unpublished material are warranted is uncertain and will vary from question to question. In deciding how extensively to search, reviewers must weigh the costs against the potential gain in information. In many cases, decisions such as this will rest on practical considerations; for example, the decision whether to include foreign language publications will often depend on the availability of someone who can assist with translations.

Selecting Studies

The selection of studies for inclusion in a meta-analysis is primarily governed by the definition of the research question. The latter needs to be clearly defined in terms of the population, the intervention or exposure, and the outcome.

For example, the research question for one recent meta-analysis (Stachenko, Bravo, Coté, Boucher, & Battista, 1991) was defined in the following terms: Does an aspirin regimen, with or without other antiplatelet drugs, prevent fatal and nonfatal stroke or cardiovascular disease mortality following transient ischemic attack in adults? The selection of studies here was based on predetermined criteria for the research design, target groups, and end points. The application of these criteria narrowed the meta-analysis to 7 clinical trials from an initial list of 19. Clearly, the choices made in this initial stage influenced the capacity to generalize the results of the meta-analysis. Balance is needed between being overly restrictive and overly inclusive.

Another step in a meta-analysis is the determination of the outcome of interest and the definition of the treatment and the intervention groups. In a meta-analysis of studies of breast-feeding (Bernard-Bonnin, Stachenko, Rousseau, & Girard, 1989), the outcome measure was defined simply as "breast-feeding for a minimum of 4 weeks, including the use of supplemental formula at a maximum of once per week." In other studies, the outcome measure may subsume multiple subcategories. For example, the aspirin study used several outcome measures: not only total cardiovascular deaths but also subcategories such as fatal myocardial infarction, sudden cardiac death, and fatal and nonfatal stroke, which represent neither mutually exclusive nor completely exhaustive subdivisions of the outcome.

Precise specification of the intervention is also important. In the aspirin study, 3 nonmutually exclusive treatment groups were defined: aspirin only, aspirin combinations, and any regimen including aspirin. It should be noted that within each there were variations in dosage, mode, frequency of administration, and compliance. This type of heterogeneity needs to be considered in interpreting the results of a meta-analysis.

The definition of control groups also requires attention. For example, in the breast-feeding study, the experimental groups were defined in terms of whether the women had early contact with their infants, restriction of feeding supplementation, and postpartum education by a nurse with or without telephone follow-up. The control group was defined by reference to the experimental group as the individuals receiving "usual care," that is, not receiving any of the experimental interventions. Because practices among hospitals vary considerably, however, the actual makeup of the control group may have differed from study to study.

Once these definitions have been established, all articles obtained must be assessed to see whether these criteria have been met. To ensure the reproducibility of these assessments, at least two reviewers should assess the relevance of each article, and agreement between them should be measured and reported using kappa (a chance corrected measure of agreement; Cohen, 1960, 1968). "Experts" in a particular area frequently have preformed opinions that can bias their assessments of both the relevance and the validity of particular articles (Cooper, 1986; Cooper & Ribble, 1989; Gotzsche, 1987; Oxman & Guyatt, submitted for publication).

Thus, while it is important that at least one reviewer be knowledgeable in the area under review, it may be an advantage to include a second one who is not an expert and therefore is without preformed opinions (Oxman & Guyatt, submitted for publication).

Some meta-analysts argue that the reviewers who make these assessments should be blind to the authors, the institution, the magnitude and direction of the results, and the journal from which the article comes by only seeing edited copies of the articles (Sacks et al., 1987). Such editing is a very time-consuming process, however, and probably not warranted given the resources required and the uncertain benefit in terms of protecting against selection bias.

Validation of Studies

No consensus exists as to how the quality of studies should be evaluated. A number of instruments have been proposed to assess this, including checklists with only three items (Chalmers, Hetherington, Elbourne, Keirse, & Enkin, 1989) or even a single item (Canadian Task Force on the Periodic Health Examination, 1979; Lawrence & Mickalide, 1987). Chalmers et al. (1981) have proposed a detailed rating scheme for clinical trials, whereby numerical scores are assigned to criteria grouped under two broad categories: quality of methods and quality of analysis. Criteria in the first category include selection process, definition of treatment regimens, quality of randomization, and blinding of patients, observers, and analysts. In the second, they include reporting of the distribution of relevant characteristics in the control and experimental groups, consideration of side effects, handling of withdrawals from the study, and appropriateness of statistical tests.

Randomization and blinding are regarded as important criteria in the assessment of study quality, according to the Chalmers scoring system. Failure to meet these two major criteria usually results in low quality scores.

Validating a system for scoring the quality of research is a formidable task because there is no gold standard. It is not surprising, therefore, that, while there are many sets of criteria available for assessing methodological quality of primary research (Canadian Task Force on the Periodic Health Examination, 1979; Chalmers et al., 1981; Chalmers et al., 1989; Feinstein & Horwitz, 1982;

Horwitz & Feinstein, 1979; Lawrence & Mickalide, 1987; Sackett, Haynes, & Tugwell, 1985), none of them has been validated, nor is there a consensus as to which is "best."

Given the importance of the validity of the research that is reviewed to the conclusions of an overview, it follows that explicit criteria should be used to assess this. If studies are ranked in order of methodological quality, and their results displayed in this order in tables and graphs, a quick visual inspection of the relationship between quality and the effects observed in each study is possible. Sensitivity analysis relative to methodological quality can also be performed.

Table 19.2 presents a summary of some general methodological criteria for the study designs most frequently encountered in primary care research. These criteria can be used to formulate specific criteria for an overview, pointing out the most important threats to validity for each type of study while not overwhelming readers or reviewers with exhaustive lists of methodological considerations.

It is desirable to have an explicit approach to summarizing the quality of each study, beyond simply adding together the scores for each individual criterion. A "weakest link" approach assumes that the overall quality of a study is equal to the lowest "score" for any one criterion. A "hierarchical" approach ranks the criteria in order of importance: Studies scoring the highest on the most important criterion are ranked highest overall; within this group, the studies scoring highest on the next most important criterion are scored highest overall; and so on. Another approach is to use subjective summaries of the individual criteria.

In addition to using ratings of study quality as possible explanations for differences in results, the extent to which the primary research has met methodological standards is important per se. For example, it may be that the evidence is consistent, but all studies are seriously flawed. In such a case, the conclusions of the overview would not be nearly as strong as if consistent results had been obtained from a series of studies in which the likelihood of bias was minimal.

Another decision to be made is whether studies with low quality scores are to be retained for further analysis or excluded from consideration altogether. For example, the meta-analysis on breast-feeding referred to above (Bernard-Bonnin et al., 1989) was carried out even though some of the studies did not use randomization or

Table 19.2 Methodological Criteria for Evaluating Primary Research Studies

Type of Study	Population	Intervention or Exposure	Outcome	Completeness
Randomized control trial	Quality of randomization	Blinding of participants	Sound outcome assessment (valid, reproducible, blinded)	Completeness of follow-up
Cohort, before-after, historical-control studies	Control for known, important confounders	Sound assessment of exposure (valid, reproducible, blinded)	Sound outcome assessment (valid, reproducible, blinded)	Completeness of follow-up
Case-control study	Matching or adjustment for known, important confounders and application of same exclusion criteria to cases and controls	Sound method of ascertaining exposure (valid, reproducible, blinded)	Sound case definition (valid, reproducible, blinded)	Completeness of ascertainment of exposure
Evaluation of diagnostic test	Representative (consecutive) sample of patients	Blinded, reproducible method of testing	Gold standard (valid, reproducible, blinded)	Completeness of data (application of test and gold standard to all subjects)

blinding. The decision to include these studies was judged to be appropriate because the experimental and control groups were found to be roughly comparable with respect to characteristics that might have influenced the outcome variable. There is clearly a trade-off between quality and quantity of information when setting a threshold for quality.

Data Extraction

This step is often the most time-consuming part of the synthesis process. As with any research project, it should be done using pretested data collection forms. At least two coders should be used and agreement between them measured and reported, as suggested above for assessments of relevance. As a rule, it is much more difficult to achieve good agreement regarding assessments of quality than it is to achieve agreement regarding relevance (Marsh & Ball, 1981; Orwin & Cordray, 1981; Stock et al., 1982). This is not surprising, given that more judgment is required for these assessments.

Given the extent of insufficient reporting in the medical literature (DerSimonian, Charette, Bucknam McPeek, & Mosteller, 1982), missing information should be obtained from investigators whenever possible. It is otherwise impossible to distinguish between what was done but not reported and what was not done. Information obtained through personal communication will strengthen an overview and often provide a valuable service to readers who are not in a position to routinely do this themselves. To avoid introducing bias, unpublished information that is obtained should be unambiguous; it should be obtained in writing; and it should be coded in the same fashion as published information, with equal regard for intercoder agreement.

Just as with assessments of relevance, the extent to which blinding is necessary in assessing methodological quality is controversial. Given the degree of judgment involved, it could be argued that blinding is more important at this stage than it is in assessing relevance; however, it is even more time-consuming to adequately edit articles so that reviewers are properly blinded. Thus, while theoretically reasonable, blinding is probably not warranted at this stage either. Sensitivity analyses around important or questionable judgments, on the other hand, can be performed relatively easily and should be done.

Data Analysis

Analysis here refers not only to the statistical analysis but to the whole process of evaluating the results of the primary research. Five possible sources of variability among studies of the same question exist: random error (chance), the methodological quality of the studies, the population, the intervention or exposure, and the outcome. The analysis should begin with a visual plot of the study results, including confidence intervals (Demets, 1987; Galbraith, 1988; Walker, Martin-Moreno, & Artalejo, 1988). If the results are extremely consistent, the search for explanations of variation can be less intense; if there is substantial variability, differences in the other four factors should be closely scrutinized to determine whether they can explain the discrepancies.

Combining results from primary research in the presence of heterogeneity is controversial. Some have argued that heterogeneity presents little problem when one is seeking to discover an overall treatment effect (Peto, 1987). At the other extreme, it has been argued that more is to be learned from a careful examination of the differences in study design associated with differences in outcome than by combining study results (Horwitz, 1987).

When differences in outcome cannot be explained by the play of chance, studies must be examined carefully for features that can explain the different results. Under these circumstances, an overall effect size, if it is calculated, must be interpreted cautiously. Similarly, inferences based on interstudy differences should be made cautiously, if at all, even when there is statistically significant heterogeneity (Oxman & Guyatt, 1992; Peto, 1987). Between-study comparisons should be viewed as hypothesis-generating analyses. Hypothesis testing based on interstudy differences is threatened both by capitalizing on chance and by confounders, and should be avoided.

Formal statistical analysis should be conducted when appropriate for essentially the same reasons as in primary analysis of data;

that is, as a tool for reducing data and avoiding errors in inferences (Cooper & Rosenthal, 1980; Pillemer, 1984). The choice of which statistical method to use is another controversial issue (Bailey, 1987; Berlin, Laird, Sacks, & Chalmers, 1989; Canner, 1987; Demets, 1987). Several established methods are available for issues of therapy or prevention where the outcome is expressed as a proportion. These include the Mantel-Haenszel technique and other estimators of the combined odds ratio (Breslow & Day, 1980; Canner, 1987; Demets, 1987; DerSimonian & Laird, 1986; Greenland, 1987; Halvorsen, 1986); logistic regression, which allows estimation of the effects of covariates such as study design or methodological quality (Breslow & Day, 1980); the DerSimonian and Laird method, which uses the risk difference; and methods for combining relative risks (DerSimonian & Laird, 1986).

If a test for heterogeneity is not statistically significant, one cannot necessarily conclude that heterogeneity does not exist, because the test used may have had limited power (Breslow & Day, 1980). Therefore, careful attention must be paid to the visual display of results, and clinical judgment must always be used in deciding which studies can be combined, irrespective of the results of tests of heterogeneity (Halvorsen, 1986).

All of the methods that are in common use based on the odds ratio assume a fixed effects model; that is, variation between studies is not included in calculations of the 95% confidence interval or the statistical significance of the common odds ratio. The effect of this is that, when there is substantial between-study variation in results, the estimate of the 95% confidence intervals is likely to be "anticonservative" (small) as compared with an estimate based on a random effects model (Bailey, 1987; Berlin, Laird, Sacks, & Chalmers, 1989). To avoid misrepresenting the level of confidence in estimates of effectiveness, when there is significant heterogeneity (say, $p \leq 0.10$), a range can be reported rather than the 95% confidence intervals, and the statistical significance of the common odds ratio should be interpreted cautiously.

Methods for combining the results of studies of therapy in which the outcome is expressed as a continuous variable have been used widely in the psychological and educational literature, in particular, in various "effect size" techniques (Cooper, 1989; Glass, McGaw, & Smith, 1981; Hedges & Olkin, 1985). These techniques have not, however, been widely used in the medical literature. The results, which are in units of standard deviations, can be difficult to interpret. Meta-analyses in which effect size techniques have been used have generated considerable controversy in the psychology literature (Pillemer, 1984). Hedges and Olkin have summarized the various techniques (Hedges & Olkin, 1985).

Reporting Results

Published guidelines exist for reporting overviews (Halvorsen, 1986; L'Abbe et al., 1987; Mulrow, 1987; Oxman & Guyatt, 1988; Sacks et al., 1987) as well as for reporting structured abstracts for overviews (Haynes, Mulrow, Huth, Altman, & Gardner, 1990). In addition to clearly reporting the methods that were used, publications should take care to make clear the clinical relevance of the overview. A "balance sheet" (Eddy, 1990) is a useful way to display the results of an overview, such as for each target population or intervention the expected outcomes with their 95% confidence intervals presented in tabular form. Table 19.3 shows an example of such a balance sheet for the use of pentamidine to prevent *Pneumocystis carinii pneumonia* in patients with AIDS. Because odds ratios can be difficult to interpret clinically, it is helpful to transform them into a more "clinically relevant" measure, such as the "number needed to treat" (Laupacis, Sackett, & Roberts, 1988), and to present the number needed to treat for the range of baseline risk of acquiring the illness that is normally encountered in clinical practice, or the attributable benefits and risks, as illustrated in the table.

It is often not practical to specify detailed criteria for deciding upon practice recommendations a priori. In general, these decisions rest upon estimates of the magnitude of the benefits, the risks and costs, the relative values (preferences) attributed to these, the precision (certainty) of the estimates, and the strength (validity) of the evidence. Some degree of judgment is inevitable in reaching a conclusion. Nonetheless, the basis of any recommendation should be clearly detailed and sufficient data provided such that it is possible for a reader to easily assess the strength of the recommendation and make an informed decision about whether to agree.

Table 19.3 Balance Sheet: Pentamidine for the Prevention of
Pneumocystis Carinii Pneumonia (PCP) in Patients with AIDS

Balance Sheet for Pentamidine (q4wk × 18 months)
(per 100 patients treated)

Baseline risk (percent)	Cases of PCP Prevented n/100 (95% CI)	Deaths Delayed n/100 (95% CI)	Withdrawals from Treatment Due to Side Effects n/100	Patients with Severe Cough n/100	Cost per 100 Patients × 18 Months* (dollars)
20	10 (5-14)	5 (5-10)	2	38	129,600
40	18 (7-26)	8 (7-17)	2	38	129,600
60	21 (8-34)	8 (8-20)	2	38	129,600
80	17 (6-31)	6 (6-16)	2	38	129,600

*Cost of pentamidine only, per patient, not including cost associated with administration or cost of nebulizer ($72/month × 18 months).

Conclusion

There is a scientific basis on which to make methodological decisions when undertaking an overview, and the same principles apply whether one is conducting a "quick and dirty" review in the context of one's clinical practice (Oxman, 1989) or preparing a formal meta-analysis. Although many of the decisions that must be made are not clear-cut, recognizing these underlying principles can help clinicians and reviewers arrive at answers that are more likely to be valid and clinically applicable and do so with greater efficiency.

Scientific investigation actively promotes uncertainty while seeking "absolute truths." Paradoxically, through its promotion of uncertainty, the application of scientific principles is the most efficient way of discovering what works and what does not. Unfortunately, medical science seldom yields "definitive" conclusions about what to do. Scientific overviews are essential for assessing the strength of the evidence underlying recommendations for care—authoritative or otherwise—and for distinguishing opinions from facts when determining how to proceed.

References

Bailey, K. R. (1987). Interstudy differences: How should they influence the interpretation and analysis of results. *Statistics and Medicine, 6*, 351-358.

Begg, C. B., & Berlin, J. A. (1989). Publication bias and dissemination of clinical research. *Journal of the National Cancer Institute, 81*, 107-115.

Berlin, J. A., Laird, N. M., Sacks, H. S., & Chalmers, T. C. (1989). A comparison of statistical methods for combining event rates from clinical trials. *Statistics and Medicine, 8*, 141-151.

Bernard-Bonnin, A. C., Stachenko, S., Rousseau, E., & Girard, G. (1989). Meta-analyse des facteurs intra-hospitaliers sur la dureé de l'allaitement. *Revue Epidémiologique et Santé Publique, 37*, 217-225.

Bernstein, F. (1988). The retrieval of randomized clinical trials in liver diseases from the medical literature: Manual versus MEDLARS searches. *Controlled Clinical Trials, 9*, 23-31.

Breslow, N. E., & Day, N. E. (1980). Combination of results from a series of 2×2 tables: Control of confounding. In *Statistical methods in cancer research: The analysis of case-control studies* (Vol. 1, pp. 136-146). Lyon, France: International Agency for Research on Cancer.

Canadian Task Force on the Periodic Health Examination. (1979). The periodic health examination. *Canadian Medical Association Journal, 121*, 3-11.

Canner, P. L. (1987). An overview of six clinical trials of aspirin in coronary heart disease. *Statistics and Medicine, 6*, 255-263.

Chalmers, I., Hetherington, J., Elbourne, D., Keirse, M. J. N. C., & Enkin, M. (1989). Materials and methods used in synthesizing evidence to evaluate the effects of care during pregnancy and childbirth. In I. Chalmers, M. Enkin, & M. J. N. C. Keirse (Eds.), *Effective care in pregnancy and childbirth* (pp. 39-66). Oxford: Oxford University Press.

Chalmers, T. C., Smith, H., Blackburn, B., Silverman, B., Schroeder, B., Reitman, D., & Ambroz, A. (1981). A method for assessing the quality of a randomized control trial. *Controlled Clinical Trials, 2*, 31-49.

Cohen, J. (1960). A coefficient of agreement for nominal scales. *Educational and Psychological Measurement, 20*, 37-46.

Cohen, J. (1968). Weighted kappa: Nominal scale agreement with provision for scaled disagreement or partial credit. *Psychological Bulletin, 70*, 213-220.

Cooper, H. (1986). On the social psychology of using research review: The case of desegregation and the black achiever. In R. S. Feldman (Ed.), *Social psychology of education* (pp. 341-363). Cambridge: Cambridge University Press.

Cooper, H., & Ribble, R. G. (1989). Influences on the outcome of literature searches for integrative research reviews. *Knowledge, 10*, 179-201.

Cooper, H. M. (1989). *Integrating research: A guide for literature reviews.* Newbury Park, CA: Sage.

Cooper, H. M., & Rosenthal, R. (1980). Statistical versus traditional procedures for summarizing research findings. *Psychological Bulletin, 124*, 711-718.

Demets, D. L. (1987). Methods for combining randomized clinical trials: Strengths and limitations. *Statistics and Medicine, 6*, 341-348.

De Neef, P. (1988). The comprehensiveness of computer-assisted searches of the medical literature. *Journal of Family Practice, 27,* 404-408.

DerSimonian, R., Charette, L. J., Bucknam McPeek, B. A., & Mosteller, F. (1982). Reporting on methods in clinical trials. *New England Journal of Medicine, 306,* 1332-1337.

DerSimonian, R., & Laird, N. (1986). Meta-analysis in clinical trials. *Controlled Clinical Trials, 7,* 177-188.

Dickerson, K., Chan, S., Chalmers, T. C., Sacks, H. S., & Smith, H. (1987). Publication bias and clinical trials. *Controlled Clinical Trials, 8,* 343-353.

Dickerson, K., Hewitt, P., Mutch, L., Chalmers, I., & Chalmers, T. C. (1985). Perusing the literature: Comparison of MEDLINE searching with a perinatal trials database. *Controlled Clinical Trials, 6,* 306-317.

Dickerson, K., Higgins, K., & Meinert, C. L. (1990). Identification of meta-analyses: The need for standard terminology. *Controlled Clinical Trials, 11,* 52-66.

Easterbrook, P. J., Berlin, J. A., Gopalan, R., & Matthews, D. R. (1991). Publication bias in clinical research. *Lancet, 337,* 867-872.

Eddy, D. M. (1990). Comparing benefits and harms: The balance sheet. *Journal of the American Medical Association, 263,* 2493-2505.

Feinstein, A. R., & Horwitz, R. I. (1982). Double standards, scientific methods, and epidemiological research. *New England Journal of Medicine, 307,* 1611-1617.

Galbraith, R. F. (1988). A note on graphical presentation of estimated odds ratios from several clinical trials. *Statistics and Medicine, 7,* 889-894.

Glass, G. V. (1976). Primary, secondary and meta-analysis of research. *Educational Researcher, 5,* 3-8.

Glass, G. V., McGaw, B., & Smith, M. L. (1981). *Meta-analysis in social research.* Beverly Hills, CA: Sage.

Gotzsche, P. C. (1987). Reference bias in reports of drug trials. *British Medical Journal, 295,* 654-656.

Greenland, S. (1987). Quantitative methods in the review of epidemiologic literature. *Epidemiological Reviews, 9,* 1-30.

Halvorsen, K. T. (1986). Combining results from independent investigations: Meta-analysis in medical research. In J. C. Bailar & F. Mosteller (Eds.), *Medical uses of statistics* (pp. 392-416). Waltham, MA: NEJM Books.

Haynes, R. B., Mulrow, C. D., Huth, E. J., Altman, D. G., & Gardner, M. J. (1990). More informative abstracts revisited. *Annals of Internal Medicine, 113,* 69-76.

Hedges, L. V., & Olkin, I. (1985). *Statistical methods for meta-analysis.* Orlando, FL: Academic Press.

Horwitz, R. I. (1987). Complexity and contradiction in clinical trial research. *American Journal of Medicine, 82,* 498-510.

Horwitz, R. I., & Feinstein, A. R. (1979). Methodological standards and contradictory results in case-control research. *American Journal of Medicine, 66,* 556-564.

Jackson, G. B. (1980). Methods for integrative reviews. *Review of Educational Research, 50,* 438-460.

Kirpalani, H., Schmidt, B., McKibbon, K. A., Haynes, R. B., & Sinclair, J. C. (1989). Searching medline for high quality studies on care of the newborn. *Pediatrics, 83,* 543-546.

L'Abbe, K. A., Detsky, A. S., & O'Rourke, K. (1987). Meta-analysis in clinical research. *Annals of Internal Medicine, 107,* 224-233.

Laupacis, A., Sackett, D. L., & Roberts, R. S. (1988). An assessment of clinically useful measures of the consequences of treatment. *New England Journal of Medicine, 318*, 1728-1733.

Lawrence, R. S., & Mickalide, A. D. (1987). Preventive services in clinical practice: Designing the periodic health examination. *Journal of the American Medical Association, 257*, 2205-2207.

Marsh, H. W., & Ball, S. (1981). Interjudgmental reliability of reviews for the *Journal of Educational Psychology*. *Journal of Educational Psychology, 73*, 872-880.

Mulrow, C. D. (1987). The medical review article: State of the science. *Annals of Internal Medicine, 106*, 485-488.

National Library of Medicine. (1989). *Medical subject headings: Annotated alphabetic list* (PB 89-100010). Washington, DC: Government Printing Office.

Nelder, J. A. (1988). Discussion of the paper by Begg and Berlin. *Journal of the Royal Statistical Society Association, 151*(3), 457.

Orwin, R. G., & Cordray, D. S. (1985). Effects of deficient reporting on meta-analysis: A conceptual framework and reanalysis. *Psychological Bulletin, 97*(1), 134-147.

Oxman, A. D. (1989). Science of reading. *Pediatrics, 83*, 617-619.

Oxman, A. D., & Guyatt, G. H. (1988). Guidelines for reading literature reviews. *Canadian Medical Association Journal, 138*, 697-703.

Oxman, A. D., & Guyatt, G. H. (1992). A consumers' guide to subgroup analyses. *Annals of Internal Medicine, 116*, 78-84.

Oxman, A. D., & Guyatt, G. H. (submitted for publication). *Expertise, training and science in review articles*. Manuscript under review.

Peto, R. (1987). Why do we need systematic overviews of randomized trials. *Statistics and Medicine, 6*, 233-240.

Pillemer, D. B. (1984). Conceptual issues in research synthesis. *Journal of Special Education, 18*, 27-40.

Poynard, T., & Conn, H. O. (1985). The retrieval of randomized clinical trials in liver disease from the medical literature. *Controlled Clinical Trials, 6*, 271-279.

Sackett, D. L., Haynes, R. B., & Tugwell, P. (1985). *Clinical epidemiology: A basic science for clinical medicine*. Boston: Little, Brown.

Sacks, H. S., Berrier, J., Reitman, D., Ancona-Berk, V. A., & Chalmers, T. C. (1987). Meta-analyses of randomized controlled trials. *New England Journal of Medicine, 316*, 450-455.

Stachenko, S., Bravo, G., Coté, R., Boucher, J., & Battista, R. (1991). Aspirin in transient ischemic heart attacks and minor stroke: A meta analysis. *Family Practice Research Journal, 11*, 179-191.

Stock, W. A., Okun, M. A., Haring, M. J., Miller, W., Kinney, C., & Ceurvorst, R. W. (1982). Rigor in data synthesis: A case study of reliability in meta-analysis. *Educational Researcher, 11*, 10-14.

Thacker, S. B. (1988). Meta-analysis: A quantitative approach to research integration. *Journal of the American Medical Association, 259*, 1685-1689.

Walker, A. M., Martin-Moreno, J. M., & Artalejo, F. R. (1988). Odd man out: A graphical approach to meta-analysis. *American Journal of Public Health, 78*, 961-966.

Yusuf, S., Simon, R., & Ellenberg, S. (1987). Proceedings of methodological issues in overviews of randomized clinical trials. *Statistics and Medicine, 6*, 217-409.

20 Options for Nurses in the Primary Care Setting

CAROL L. McWILLIAM

The assessment of nursing interventions presents a complex challenge for practitioners and researchers alike. Assessment of the effectiveness of concrete tasks, such as teaching about immunization, monitoring vital signs, or ensuring medication compliance, can be readily handled through surveys, clinical trials, and other quantitative methods that can measure immediate outcomes. But much of the significance of family practice nursing is contained within the caring relationship between nurse and patient—the provision of continuous nurturing, support, and guidance to a wide variety of patients and their family caregivers, including parents of children with chronic health problems, new parents, and those caring for aging patients. Such intervention is not easily quantified, for it must be ongoing, affective, responsive to unique human needs, and often intuitive. In short, the essence of caring calls for a qualitative approach to assessing its effectiveness.

Alternatives for Assessing Family Practice Nursing Care

Two alternatives provide sound but as yet infrequently used strategies for primary care nurses seeking to assess their efforts: *interpretive research* using a phenomenological approach and *action research*. Each lends itself to a particular kind of research question.

Interpretive Research

The interpretive researcher operates with a different worldview than that of the traditional scientific researcher. The topic of concern is human experience, which is believed to be socially created, subjectively perceived, and unique to the individuals, time, and place being studied. The researcher seeks to understand dynamic human relationships, feelings, thoughts, and behaviors, which undergo constant change as experience unfolds. This purpose contrasts sharply with the traditional search for facts about cause-and-effect linear relationships between carefully singled out variables under rigorously controlled conditions (Lincoln & Guba, 1985; Patton, 1990).

While there are several theoretical approaches to undertaking interpretive research, a particularly useful structure for assessing primary care intervention is phenomenology. The central research question addressed in phenomenological research is this: "What is the structure and essence of the experience of this phenomenon for these people?" (Patton, 1990, p. 88).

The guiding principles (Spiegelberg, 1976) of this type of analysis are straightforward. Simply stated, the process begins with a commitment to investigating a particular phenomenon—such as a nursing intervention—and attempting to discover its minute particulars. Who and what were involved? When, where, why, and how did the experience unfold? What did the phenomenon mean to each person who experienced it? The general patterns and themes that have occurred are then identified, and the researcher and the research participants attempt to understand together what is happening and what it has meant for all involved. They consciously question their understanding and ultimately decide how they might interpret the meaning of the experience under study.

PRACTICAL APPLICATIONS

Phenomenological research seeks understanding of a process, and nursing intervention is, above all, a process. Hence many research questions relevant to assessing nursing intervention may be studied using this approach. Examples of such questions include the following: How do parents experience the nurse's approach to providing well-baby care (such as physical checkups, immunization updates, and ongoing guidance about parenting)? What meaning does the nurse's involvement in routine office visits have for pregnant women? How do diabetic patients experience the nurse's approach to monitoring their weight, dietary intake, blood and urine test results, and all of the related teaching?

Answers to these questions would provide information about intervention *processes* rather than outcomes. Knowing whether parents were finding their approaches to providing well-baby care as supportive and helpful, or as intimidating and overwhelming, could help the individual nurse adjust his or her approach if and as necessary. (Findings may suggest that increasing the emphasis on the nurse's nurturing and supportive roles, and modifying the teaching component, might enhance effectiveness in this area.) Similarly, if it were determined that pregnant women find the nurse's empathic understanding about their experiences of physiological changes to be a helpful component of routine office visits, primary care physician-nurse teams might modify their respective roles during these visits. And, in the third scenario, a detailed picture of diabetic patients undergoing regular checkups may provide helpful insights about how the nurse may help the patient feel more of an equal partner in control of the monitoring process.

These scenarios are hypothetical, for phenomenological research of this nature has not yet taken hold in assessing interventions in office-based primary care; however, nurses in several other settings have used this methodology successfully. For examples, the reader may wish to review Benner's (1984) analysis of what expert nurses do in specific patient care situations, Drew's (1986) study of patient experiences with caregivers, Andre's study (reported in Parse, Coyne, & Smith, 1985) of "reaching out" as part of the helping relationship, Banonis's (1989) study of the experience of recovering from addiction, Geissler's (1990) study of nurturance, and Davies and Oberle's (1990) study of the supportive role of palliative care nurses.

My own phenomenological research to assess intervention began with a pilot project undertaken by a multidisciplinary team of primary care providers to describe the discharge experience of elderly patients sent home from hospital with continuing care needs (McWilliam, in press). To obtain a more in-depth understanding of factors other than diagnosis and treatment that facilitated or impeded discharge from hospital and adequacy of care at home, the experiences of 12 patients and their family caregivers and of 62 health professionals were documented. A 6-week period of data collection included a review of charts and home care records, observations of discharge planning conferences and actual discharge incidents, and in-depth interviews conducted in both the hospital and the home settings. Inductive analysis and interpretation were carried out concurrently and extended 11 weeks beyond the data collection period. Findings illustrated the roles played by the patients' own mind-sets and family relationships in terms of the timing of their discharges and the adequacy of postdischarge care. As well, findings pinpointed interdisciplinary communication and coordination challenges and a general need of professionals and the public alike for more education about the discharge process and the home care system. The need for more involvement of the bedside nurse in in-hospital preparation of the patient for discharge, and more active participation of the family physician in community-based postdischarge care, also became very apparent. Such findings led to several concrete recommendations for improving the intervention efforts of the multidisciplinary health team.

PRACTICE IMPLICATIONS

Perhaps the biggest challenge of using phenomenology to assess primary care intervention is the time, effort, and skill required to collect and analyze data. Appropriate methods include observation, in-depth interview, and document review (Patton, 1990). For overviews of these methods, the reader is referred to Volume 2 of the Research Methods for Primary Care series (Stewart, Tudiver, Bass, Dunn, & Norton, 1992): Morgan (Chapter 15, "Designing Focus Group Research"); Miller and Crabtree (Chapter 16, "Depth Interviewing: The Long Interview Approach"); and Crabtree (Chapter 17, "The Analysis of Narratives from a Long Interview"). Volume 3 of the same series (Crabtree & Miller, 1992) also provides a comprehensive approach to the application of qualitative methodology to primary care research. In all of the examples given, all three of these methods used in combination would achieve the greatest understanding of the process being assessed, for the actual lived experience contains data appropriate to each of these three methods.

Time and effort demands are obviously heavy. Practically speaking, it might be necessary for nurses to choose between being involved in the actual delivery of the intervention and calling on colleagues to carry out the research component, or doing the research themselves by studying the experiences of others and extracting what might be applicable to their own practice as well as that of other nurses.

To undertake phenomenological research, one needs knowledge and expertise in interpretive research methods. Many excellent references on sampling, data collection techniques, and data analysis are available. Much of this literature contains terminology that may appear jargonistic to readers without course work in the area, which can be discouraging; for such readers, Patton (1990) and Reason and Rowan (1981) afford particularly clear and practical direction. In any case, interpretive research requires intuition, analytic thinking skills, the ability to synthesize concepts, both critical and creative thinking skills, and a preparedness to spend considerable time reflecting on the topic of interest. Practice, not just theoretical mastery, is key to refining such skills.

Despite these demands, there are decided practice advantages to nurses themselves acting as the researchers. Both data collection and analysis permit—and, indeed, require—active and extensive involvement in understanding the patient. The interpretive researcher must explore the patient's personal background, situation, and ongoing concerns for, even if one does not share the patient's meanings, they do enable one as a practitioner to share the patient's experience and thereby to provide better care. Furthermore, the concern expressed and conveyed to the patient through qualitative data collection itself constitutes very individualized care (Benner & Wrubel, 1982). That is, the mere process of assessing an intervention can contribute to refining it.

Where employment circumstances dictate, or where the nurse prefers to provide concretely planned patient care and, simultaneously, to do research to assess that intervention, another exciting alternative exists: action research.

Action Research

Action research methodology has served various disciplines since its genesis in the late 1940s (Lewin, 1947) but has not been extensively employed by nurses (Hunt, 1987; Sheehan, 1990; Webb, 1989). This limited use perhaps stems more from the nursing profession's lack of contact with traditional scientists than from any lack of applicability to the field. Action research merely means using scientific methods to assess and analyze a situation, to plan and implement appropriate action, and then to reassess, reanalyze, or evaluate the action taken. The evaluation stage then leads to a repetition of this whole cycle of activities. The parallels with the nursing process are striking.

The central purpose of action research is to study processes through changing them and seeing the effect (Sanford, 1990). Furthermore, the approach involves both researchers and research participants (the "subjects" of traditional research), who work together throughout each step in the cycle. The general research question is this: How can we further refine this process through the efforts of all participants?

We all use the basic steps of action research when we solve any practical problem or learn any skill; we do this, however, without formalizing the research component inherent in it. By formalizing the research component, we consciously obtain and document knowledge of the effect of our everyday experiences and thereby create a concrete means of assessing intervention. Rethinking past practice leads to theoretical reformulation, which in turn leads to improved practice. The processes of rethinking both theory and practice strengthen each (Whyte, Greenwood, & Lazes, 1991).

PRACTICAL APPLICATIONS

Many questions on primary care nursing intervention may be addressed through the use of action research. For instance: How can we refine parenting classes to better meet the needs of participants? How can we improve nursing care to effect greater and more long-term success for obese patients attempting to achieve and maintain a healthier body weight? How can family practice nurses help patients to promote their own health?

Once again, answers to questions of this nature provide information about processes rather than outcomes. Research findings in each instance will include detailed data from both patients and nurses about motives, expectations, and current needs as well as valuable information about intervention approaches. Most important, the research process engages both nurses and patients in designing and testing new or refined intervention strategies. Involving our patients as research participants ensures that any refinement to our interventions are patient centered, premised upon *their* perceptions of their needs rather than upon our own directions, which are often pursued from textbook generalizations.

As with interpretive research, the value of using action research to assess nursing intervention extends beyond its potential for producing helpful research findings. The two-way intercommunication that is so much a part of the process can itself improve intervention by enhancing the relationship between nurse and patient, through confirming and solidifying in the patient's mind the notion of a shared partnership rather than a hierarchical relationship. Second, participation in the research project becomes a means of raising the patient's consciousness about health and his or her individual responsibility for it. Third, the interactive, mutually shared approach to acquiring data allows the nurse to gain a more in-depth appreciation of the patient's world—the nurse-researcher and the patient participant educate each other (Freire, 1976). Finally, nurses can refine their practice by merely undertaking the research, for the act of research requires that one engage in "reflection-in-action," a conscious, continuous process of mental assessment of effort, which provides a basis for constantly improving practice (Russell, 1987).

Personally, I am just beginning some very exciting action research (Deagle & McWilliam, 1991) to assess a health promotion intervention strategy. This project has been designed as a collaborative team effort in which a family physician and a nurse will work with a group of rural farmers concerned about the potential health hazards of the herbicides they apply to their crops. Together, we will help participants to assess the potential risks and to make group decisions on any actions to be taken. This process will include testing of well water and soil to measure contamination levels; facilitated group discussion with experts (e.g., toxicologists, environmentalists); facilitated group exploration of the resources available, the value trade-offs to be considered, and the limitations to achieving any potential solutions; and facilitated group decision making to effect a consensus about action to be taken, if any. We will qualitatively document this entire process and use inductive analysis to uncover a more in-depth understanding of health promotion as a process. Once the group decides on a direction, we will qualitatively study all relevant health behaviors and farming practices for a one-year period. At the end of that time frame, we will meet with participants again so that together we can assess, both quantitatively and qualitatively, the effectiveness of this whole health promotion intervention. In this way, action research will allow us to *do* health promotion and, at the same time, will give us a better understanding of the meaning of health and health promotion to guide future efforts, whether with individual patients in the office or with groups of people in the community.

PRACTICE IMPLICATIONS

The methods of action research may combine quantitative with qualitative approaches or may be solely qualitative in nature. Several useful references may help in the project design phase (Randall, 1981; Torbert, 1981; Whyte et al., 1991). The practicing nurse may accomplish qualitative data collection by involving groups of patients in a series of sessions to assess, plan, implement, and evaluate the intervention under investigation, whether in parenting groups, weight loss counseling sessions, or a series of health promotion seminars. Alternatively, the process may be conducted with a number of individual patients over a prolonged period of time. With the written consent of participants, sessions may be audio- or videotaped as a means of data collection. The nurse-researcher would then analyze the content of these tapes, searching for common themes and patterns; confirm the findings with participants; and involve them in making recommendations for refinement of the intervention process. Documenting and reporting findings complete the research activity.

Practically speaking, action research has one outstanding advantage. Designing a study, implementing data collection, and evaluating the intervention all readily integrate into the practice nurse's role of providing care; only the analysis and dissemination of research results would be above and beyond her or his usual commitments. Thus action research is cost-efficient. The office nurse can therefore more readily justify this allocation of resources to health care system administrators concerned about economic constraints.

A key disadvantage to be overcome, however, is that hard-nosed "traditional scientists" may reject action research as simple story-telling, unworthy of scientific merit. Hence nurses who choose this approach to assessing intervention will have to present a strong case. It can be argued that, if one can accept the numbers that measure the perceptions and attitudes that have arisen in response to an intervention, then surely the data that reflect the actual intervention cannot be scientifically inferior (Whyte et al., 1991). Action research collects live data on the intervention process itself and is thus invaluable in assessing the nurse's role.

Conclusion

"Experience rooted in systematic study and in actual clinical practice is the crucial element in the development of clinical knowledge" (Benner & Wrubel, 1982). Nurses have been overly constrained by the stringent requirements of formal theories developed in the tradition of classical seventeenth-century science, which embodies an atomistic, mechanistic view of the person. People, and the very human process of caring for them, cannot be considered machinelike, orderly, predictable, concretely observable, and measurable. Human issues, which are shaped by the meaning assigned by people who actually experience these issues and by the context within which they are experienced, are central to expert nursing care (Benner, 1984).

Assessing an intervention when that intervention is an ongoing, dynamic, human process presents nurses with a unique research challenge. Each of the two approaches that can meet this challenge—phenomenology and action research—has advantages. Each makes research an integral part of practice; each focuses on the essence of a process, which is what nursing is; and each enables nurses engaged in providing primary care to explore, to describe, and ultimately to assess their greatest intervention: nursing care.

References

Banonis, B. (1989). The lived experience of recovering from addiction: A phenomenological study. *Nursing Science Quarterly, 2*, 37-43.

Benner, P. (1984). *From novice to expert: Excellence and power in clinical nursing practice.* Menlo Park, CA: Addison-Wesley.

Benner, P., & Wrubel, J. (1982). Skilled clinical knowledge: The value of perceptual awareness. *Nurse Educator, 7*(3), 1117.

Crabtree, B., & Miller, W. (Eds.). (1992). *Research methods for primary care: Vol. 3. Doing qualitative research in primary care: Multiple strategies.* Newbury Park, CA: Sage.

Davies, B., & Oberle, K. (1990). Dimensions of the supportive role of the nurse in palliative care. *Oncology Nursing Forum, 17*(1), 87-94.

Deagle, G., & McWilliam, C. (1991). Health promotion action research: Addressing well-water contamination in Caradoc Township. In F. Tudiver, M. J. Bass, E. V. Dunn, P. G. Norton, & M. Stewart (Eds.), *Proceedings of foundations of primary care research: Assessing interventions in primary care.* Toronto: University of Toronto and University of Western Ontario.

Drew, N. (1986). Exclusion and confirmation: A phenomenology study of patients' experiences with caregivers. *Image: Journal of Nursing Scholarship, 18*, 39-43.

Freire, P. (1976). *Education: The practice of freedom.* London: Writers and Readers Publishing Cooperative.

Geissler, E. (1990). An exploratory study of selected female registered nurses: Meaning and expression of nurturance. *Journal of Advanced Nursing, 15*, 525-530.

Hunt, M. (1987). The process of translating research findings into nursing practice. *Journal of Advanced Nursing, 12*, 101-110.

Lewin, K. (1947). Group decision and social change. In T. M. Newcomb & E. L. Hartley (Eds.), *Readings in social psychology.* New York: Holt, Rinehart & Winston.

Lincoln, Y., & Guba, E. (1985). *Naturalistic inquiry.* Beverly Hills, CA: Sage.

McWilliam, C. (in press). From hospital to home. *Family Medicine.*

Parse, R. R., Coyne, A. B., & Smith, M. J. (1985). *Nursing research: Qualitative methods.* Bowie, MD: Brady Communications.

Patton, M. (1990). *Qualitative evaluation and research methods* (2nd ed.). Newbury Park, CA: Sage.

Randall, R. (1981). Doing dialogical research. In P. Reason & J. Rowan (Eds.), *Human inquiry: A sourcebook of new paradigm research* (pp. 349-361). Toronto: John Wiley.

Reason, P., & Rowan, J. (Eds.). (1981). *Human inquiry: A sourcebook of new paradigm research.* New York: John Wiley.

Russell, T. (1987). Reflection-in action: A new perspective on teachers' work. *The Canadian Administrator, 26*(6), 2-4.

Sanford, N. (1990). A model for action research. In P. Reason & J. Rowan (Eds.), *Human inquiry: A sourcebook of new paradigm research* (pp. 173-181). Toronto: John Wiley.

Sheehan, J. (1990). Investigating change in a nursing context. *Journal of Advanced Nursing, 15,* 819-824.

Spiegelberg, H. (1976). *The phenomenological movement* (Vols. 1, 2). The Hague, the Netherlands: Martinus Nijhoff.

Stewart, M., Tudiver, F., Bass, M. J., Dunn, E. V., & Norton, P. G. (Eds.). (1992). *Research methods for primary care: Vol. 2. Tools for primary care research.* Newbury Park, CA: Sage.

Torbert, W. (1981). Empirical, behavioural, theoretical, and attentional skills necessary for collaborative inquiry. In P. Reason & J. Rowan (Eds.), *Human inquiry: A sourcebook of new paradigm research* (pp. 437-446). Toronto: John Wiley.

Webb, C. (1989). Action research: Philosophy, methods, and personal experiences. *Journal of Advanced Nursing, 14,* 403-410.

Whyte, W. F., Greenwood, D. J., & Lazes, P. (1991). Participatory action research: Through practice to science in social research. In W. F. Whyte (Ed.), *Participatory action research* (pp. 19-55). Newbury Park, CA: Sage.

PART IV

Primary Care Interventions
in the Future

The closing chapter of the volume presents four panelists, Drs. Bain, Bass, Labrecque, and Seifert, discussing what each views as the most important aspects of primary care to be assessed in the future. Their ideas and their exchange with the audience shed light on several key issues, in particular, continuity of care and the need to define a focus in primary care research.

21 Assessing Interventions in Primary Care in the Future

JOHN BAIN
MARTIN J. BASS
RICHARD GLAZIER
MICHEL LABRECQUE
MILTON H. SEIFERT, JR.
FRED TUDIVER
EARL V. DUNN

As the final summary for this volume, we asked four experienced primary care researchers (three academic family physicians and one community practitioner) to discuss the topic: "assessing interventions in primary care in the future." Specifically, we wanted to know what the panelists believed should be the content of research in primary care and upon what it should be focused. The discussion was then opened to an audience consisting of more than 80 researchers in the field.

Of the panelists, Dr. Bass discussed four content areas that need attention: high-risk individuals, enhancing health, conducting effective continuing medical education, and the incorporation of appropriate technologies into clinical practice. Dr. Bain reminded the audience to retain old, established values while working with problems and new approaches, such as studying secondary prevention using a practice- and population-based approach. Dr. Seifert offered some suggestions, using entertaining anecdotes, about his approach to using patients and office staff as research collaborators. And Dr. Labrecque reminded the audience of the problem of diminishing resources for primary care research in the future.

The panel was chaired by Dr. Richard Glazier, an academic family physician. Dr. Earl Dunn helped with the transcriptions of the session so that they could be presented in this book.

A lively discussion with the audience followed the introductory remarks by each panelist. Of the several key issues discussed, one was continuity of care, on which there seemed to be agreement that it is an important topic but one difficult to study. The remainder of the time was spent discussing the issue of focus in primary care research, which emerged as a rather vigorous exchange of views on the definition of focusing and its pros and cons. For many, the wish seems not to be for becoming reductionists, as is the case in traditional biomedical research, but for becoming *multifocused*—an idea that may be innovative and comfortable for primary care providers. This last part of the session was most exciting; it is where the group started to describe a new paradigm for the "environ-ment" of primary care research in the future.

DR. RICHARD GLAZIER: Today we have four panelists: Martin Bass from the University of Western Ontario; John Bain from Southamp-ton, England; Milton Seifert, a community family physician from Excelsior, Minnesota; and Michel Labrecque from Laval University, Quebec City. Each of our panelists, with some audience input, will contribute to the discussion of several key topics related to assessing interventions in the future: most significantly, the content of primary care research, and the need to be focused in our research and what that means.

DR. MARTIN BASS: Until now, the content of intervention assessments in primary care has been the clinical therapies we use and what happens in the practice setting. I would like to identify four other places where we have to put some attention. The first is the early detection of those who are high risk for the social and psychological problems that are so difficult to treat—for example, spousal abuse or problems with alcohol. Research is needed on how to help these persons avoid the full-blown manifestations of the problem. The second area is to look at enhancing health. The WHO definition of health is that health can be seen as a resource for living. Family doctors say that they are interested in pursuing this view of health, but I don't think that they yet have the skills. We have to develop those skills and then assess them. The third area is making an impact on the care given by the physician—how to provide effective continuing medical education. The fourth is an area of my personal interest: the incorporation of appropriate technology into practice so that both doctors and patients benefit.

DR. JOHN BAIN: I'd like to discuss the concept of "back to the future." Roberts, in his book *History of the World* [1976] stated in his concluding paragraph that "only two general truths emerge from the study of history—one is that things tend to change much more, and more quickly, than one might think. The other is that they tend to change much less and much more slowly than one might think." The difficulty is that at any moment in history we cannot predict which direction it will go. When making predictions about the future, I always feel somewhat uncomfortable. Even in my short lifetime, there have been things that have happened in primary care that I would never have predicted.

My thoughts include "something old" and "something new." There are three things that are old that will always remain with us, whether we are practicing clinicians, researchers, or teachers. First, the most important thing for family physicians is "being there." Maybe they are not rewarded enough for it, but it is very important that patients know they have access to us. The second thing is "doing to." We do things for our patients, which include listening and taking specific actions such as prescribing and ordering investigations. Third, we prepare for patient care, which includes continuing education, and research. These old established values—being there, doing to, and preparing for—will always remain.

So what is going to be new? There will always be the balance between the person and the population, but the population-based approach is one that is increasingly going to be thrust upon us. It will be thrust upon us by patients because the extent of medical knowledge will be such that groups of patients will require collaborative care. We have had examples in some of the research efforts we have heard about here: patients with chronic illness, widowers, and so on. They seem to get support and, at times, to function better when they are looked after in groups. Patients will demand not only personal care but they will require some form of group care.

Primary prevention is a buzzword of the 1990s, but secondary prevention has to be equally important. We assume that someone will look after people with chronic illness, but how can we best provide for them? In the population-based approach, groups of health care professionals will have to learn how to work better together. I am sorry to say, one of the major blocks to providing care and interventions in terms of research and development appears to be the inability of many groups of health care professionals to work together. Skills in teamwork and team building will be an integral part of primary care in the 1990s, and research into delivery of care will have to include that provided by multiprofessional groups. Is shared care a myth or reality?

DR. MILTON SEIFERT: When I went to bed last night I had a dream. An angel appeared to me and said, "What are you going to do about the panel?" I replied, "I don't know. What do you think?" The angel suggested, "How about doing an agenda for the year 2001?" I said go ahead, write it up and take it down to the business office on the fourth floor. After lunch they had typed up a summary report of the annual meeting of the Foundations of Primary Care Research for February 14, 2001. The attendees included 100 academic physicians, 300 community physicians, 300 patients, and 500 employers, the current purchasers of care. The keynote address on strategies for designing quality assurance in health care was given by Dr. Edward Demming, now 99 years old.

Several papers were presented, including the following: an assessment of the quality of the doctor-patient relationship before rendering care, and a study of malpractice problems arising from patients failing to communicate how they feel about their illness and physicians failing to communicate how they feel about the patient. The last was given by the chair of the research committee of the association of patient advisory councils. Other papers presented by a team of doctors, patients, and employers including a doctor from Excelsior, included the value of measuring expressed emotion in the teaching of life management skills; good examples of bad research (studies that were not focused on health care improvement); designing a therapeutic community in the workplace using data from a primary care medical setting; measuring illness outcomes and health outcomes and recognizing the difference; the meta-analysis of patient-maintained medical records; and the world's best outcome measurement for primary care medical studies.

The conference included several workshops. There was one for patients, academic physicians, and community physicians involved in designing quality assessment research using the consensus manual on primary care research methodology (now in its third edition). There was one for patients on developing a research question in the practice setting—by now our patients are asking research questions. Another workshop dealt with the collaboration of doctors, patients, and employers—the new health system organizational paradigm.

Several awards were given out. There were patient awards for the best research question of 2001 and for the best method of telling the patient's story. That is the report from the 2001 Foundations conference.

AUDIENCE: I have been wondering about the definition of primary care research. I have mentioned it to a number of people. It stretches beyond community-based research and beyond family practice-based research—perhaps it is best defined as community-based team research. Team research could become our strength. Like Dr. Seifert, I also had a dream. In the year 2001, I see the World Health Organization in Geneva staffed not by a director general with a predominantly biomedical orientation but by a multidisciplinary team including a patient.

DR. MILTON SEIFERT: Perfect. I'll buy that.

AUDIENCE: May I ask one question about continuity of care of chronic illness. From some of the data coming out of Manitoba, it seems to me that it is a very difficult area to research in terms of future interventions. I wonder whether the panel feels that we should wait for the grass-roots general practitioners to start looking at it, or is it reasonable for grass-roots doctors to look to the academic centers to be setting up networks to help coordinate? A lot of energy has to be put into the system before we can get useful information that can guide our clinical practice.

DR. MILTON SEIFERT: In every paper and report that has been written about family medicine, continuity of care has always been one of the most important factors. This gets back to the idea that we haven't researched our core beliefs about comprehensive and continuing care. A family practice is too busy to mount this research on its own. One of the things about practice research is that it should not interfere with the everyday productivity of the practice. It is going to take a research team composed of a researcher, the practitioner, the patient, and the office staff all to be in on the design.

DR. JOHN BAIN: A colleague of mine has been looking at continuity of care, and one of the problems that he faces is that it could take up to 10 years of outcome measurements to assess how patients progress. It may be a belief system, but within the world of practice it varies enormously for both patients and providers. There are groups of patients who both wish and benefit from it, but there are other groups of patients who don't wish and don't necessarily benefit from it. Many patients want quick access, a quick fix, and then to get on with life. In many circumstances, that may actually be appropriate. There are other patients with chronic illness where the word is consistency of care rather than continuity of care. There is good evidence from our work in asthma, for example, that there has been lots of continuity of care, but the outcome in terms of health of the patient has not always been particularly good. What we have tried to do is to shift to consistency of care, where there is an actual planned approach for chronic illness. The assumption that continuity is good overall is one we have to question, because a doctor can sit for years and listen to the patient but that patient actually may be getting worse. A balance between continuity and consistency is what I would try to accomplish. Consistency is an important part of what we are attempting to do, but who actually benefits most from it? There is some evidence that it is actually the doctor who likes it as much as the patient. It is comfortable but it may not always be in the patient's best interest.

DR. MICHEL LABRECQUE: Research is a matter of resources. There are two types of resources. First, we need human resources. As our discipline expands, we will have more academic researchers in family medicine. The most important thing will be that more family physicians will be inspired to do research. This will drive the main human resource needs for primary care research. All residents will be trained in research, and thus we will have more links between university and community researchers. Second, we need funding. Unfortunately, we will have to cut the pie in too many pieces, so there won't be more money for individuals who are doing research. At the same time, we will see more people who are not involved in primary care who will slide into primary care research. They will go where the money is. More epidemiologists will be going into primary care research because there will be more funding. We will have more researchers in primary care and the methods will be more refined and more appropriate to primary care questions. There will be more efficient use of resources and more practice-based research, which will require minimal funding. The answers must have an impact on daily practice.

AUDIENCE: I would like to comment on something that Martin Bass alluded to, and John Bain commented on this earlier—our focus or lack of it. If we are going to contribute, we have to become more focused. Very few of us do that. It is even worse; there are a small number of people whom many of us could name who are family physicians but who have become focused. Many of these people who have contributed internationally don't show up at family practice meetings. I believe one of the reasons is that we are uncomfortable with those who become focused even in the primary care area, and we don't make them comfortable. We have to look at ourselves, our organizations, and the research we do and make sure that in our way we do become focused. We should pick a topic—for example, doctor-patient interactions or behavior changes—and stay with it for a period of time so that we know our subject, and so that researchers around the world get to know what we are doing. Most of us are not doing this.

DR. MARTIN BASS: We heard today and yesterday how family physicians can be unfocused. I don't think they are *unfocused*: family physicians and even family practice nurses are *multifocused*. The thing that we have not done well is to stay with a focus long enough. It was beautiful to hear John Bain present his otitis media studies, and to see how one study built on the previous one. I would hope that someone in Michel Labrecque's department will continue their work with warts. They know there how to assess warts, they know diagnostic instrumentation, they even know how to enroll patients who have warts. They are in a position to make major advances in that research. The same goes for Fred Tudiver with his research on widowers. He knows a lot about the assessment of widowers and how to identify specific areas of concern.

I sit on several granting committees. One of them is very biomedical in its orientation. I am struck by how they assess whether a person has the lab that can deliver what he says he is going to do. If he has the equipment for and has worked with hamsters, that doesn't necessarily mean he can do work with mice, and the reviewers become quite skeptical. I appreciated this particularly in Rebecca Henry's session. She talked about the details of the instruments and how it is really important to get to know the strengths and weaknesses of the parameters that you are working with. It may take a year and a half to develop an instrument that meets your needs; it seems inefficient to spend all that time and then walk away from the subject. The real

rewards come if you can keep building on that area. There is the mis-
apprehension that by focusing you are becoming somehow narrow.
Focusing means that you need to stay with a theme for a while, but
that doesn't mean forever. If you really believe in developmental
theory then you will become a mentor and people will build up
around you and work with you. I would hope that more of those kind
of groups will be built within family practice research.

DR. JOHN BAIN: Sometimes the problem is being too multifocused,
with an enormous breadth of activity. That is a strength of primary
care, but in some ways it is also a weakness. This is back to what is
and always will be very difficult in research—the balance between
mission-oriented research, which is at the sharp end of developing
new methods, and reality-based research, which has to do with the
family doctor, his or her support staff, and their day-to-day work.
There is a difficult balance there, and that focus needs a variety of
lenses. The important thing is to have a good idea of which lens to
use in attempting to answer a research question.

DR. MILTON SEIFERT: I would like to comment as well. The deeper
meaning of what you are saying is that we need to develop community. The thing that I liked so much about coming here was to see your
long-term comprehensive agenda for family practice research methodology. In a community it is all about mutual support and mentor-
ing. We have to appoint a committee of people who will see what
needs to be done to enhance community, community functions, and
teamwork. It does fly in the face of this part about doctors being a
little too independent, but family doctors are trying to form teams.

AUDIENCE: I am nervous about the possible misinterpretation of focusing as being interpreted as specializing. The kinds of focus we need
are on those things that are our expertise as generalists. By the year
2001, if we are all family doctors with a special interest in sports
medicine or emergency room or geriatrics, there will be no generalists
left in the system. In reflecting back, I really felt that the focus of these
conferences was the future for primary care, and that we should be
leading. We have to lead in the expertise of generalism, and not get
subdivided and end up with no generalists in the next century.

DR. MARTIN BASS: The last thing I would like to do is make the speaker
nervous—he is driving me back home! But let me say that there are
different ways of focusing. I was just thinking now about the studies
that I referred to, the wart study and the widowers study. A focus

might be on self-help groups, not necessarily for one specific topic but the approach of using self-help groups as part of our therapeutic regimens. It might be on the common treatment of skin disorders, as Michel [Labrecque] might take it, staying with a theme. Thematic focusing might be how to reflect the particular orientation and philosophy of family medicine.

DR. MILTON SEIFERT: I would like to give you all permission to remain nervous. I see a lot more harm caused by people becoming unnervous and complacent and satisfied. The American Academy of Family Practice's research data base has only 20% of research in areas that would be considered general medicine. Feel free to stay nervous and to keep thinking about it.

DR. MICHEL LABRECQUE: This is the situation, whether you like it or not. Unfortunately, general practice is moving slowly to subspecialty focusing on certain aspects of primary care but with a family practice approach. I would think it is still primary care and it will lead to opportunities to do more focused research.

DR. JOHN BAIN: I wax and wane on that question, and it is quite an important one. There are two sides to it. I have spent quite a lot of time in the last year meeting family doctors in my country who are having a difficult time because they have got a new contract, and it was a hard job before the new contract. What we need to remember is the fatiguing effect of being a family doctor for 20 years or more. There is good evidence, especially from John Howie's work in Scotland, that the stress of being a doctor is something that we haven't looked at enough. How do family doctors cope with this stress? They very often do it by having other interests within medicine. They may have a special interest in research, they may teach, they may have an interest in sports medicine, they may have an interest outside the practice. It does seem to be that those who flourish have got something in addition to concentrating on patient care alone. We are all aware of isolation and how refreshing it can be to meet with our peers and share experiences and ideas. The other side of this is that we seem to be selecting medical students from a rather narrow range of ability. If this process continues, it may be very difficult for many graduates to move into a generalized subject such as family practice. The grass roots of our discipline may be down beyond what we actually start with in residency training to whom we choose to be medical students. I hope that we, as a discipline, can influence the input to our medical schools.

AUDIENCE: I was very impressed by Dr. Bain's comment that delivering primary care is a matter of teamwork. We should complement the reductive thinkers with some inductive thinkers, of whom there are many among other health disciplines including patients and clients.

Summary

DR. FRED TUDIVER

It is interesting to hear how congruous each panelist is, despite their varied backgrounds and areas of interest. I believe the original question was addressed by each, but that each provided his or her own agenda items.

It was fascinating to see how quickly and thoroughly the researchers picked up on the topic of *focus*. I am reminded of Peter Norton's statement in Volume 1 of this series: "We are generalists, and practice in that condition. We must allow our generalist skills to carry over into our research agenda" [Norton, Stewart, Tudiver, Bass, & Dunn, 1991, p. 219]. Yet, promotion and tenure committees, grant review committees, and our reductionist specialist colleagues are always telling us to be more focused. I think each discussant of the topic of focus was talking of the need for primary care to focus *horizontally* instead of in the usual *vertical* reductionist direction. This means focusing on breadth of activity, on themes, on teamwork, or on multiple topics—all of which are unique to primary care. This is the stuff of primary care, so why not nurture it as our own?

Finally, I think Dr. Seifert's words nicely sum it up: "Feel free to stay nervous and keep thinking about it." Let us not remain complacent in this field; there is a lot of innovative work to be done, and we already have many good ideas.

References

Norton, P., Stewart, M., Tudiver, F., Bass, M. J., & Dunn, E. V. (Eds.). (1991). *Primary care research: Traditional and innovative approaches*. Newbury Park, CA: Sage.
Roberts, J. M. (1976). *History of the world*. London: Hutchinson.

Index

About the Authors

John Bain is a graduate of the University of Aberdeen, U.K., and was formerly a general practitioner in Livingston New Town in Scotland. Between 1980 and 1991, he was Chairman of the Department of Primary Medical Care at the University of Southampton and is currently conducting a project on medical audit in primary care. He is about to take the post of Chairman of the Department of General Practice at the University of Dundee. His research interests have included the study of the natural history and treatment of respiratory illness and the role of paramedical staff in general practice. In recent years, he has been involved in studying the effects of the National Health Service Reforms in the United Kingdom on the delivery of primary medical care. The creation of a new contract for general practitioners has posed a number of questions about methods of conducting performance review, and his most recent publications have focused on ways and means of developing appropriate methods for assessing general practice care.

Martin J. Bass (MD, MSc, FCFF) is Professor of Family Medicine and Epidemiology at The University of Western Ontario. He is Director of the Centre for Studies in Family Medicine and conducts research on preventive care, appropriate technology for family practice, and quality of care. He has a special interest in refining research methods for the family practice setting.

Charlyn Black (M.D., Sc.D.) is Assistant Professor in the Department of Community Health Sciences, Faculty of Medicine at the

237

University of Manitoba, and a member of the Manitoba Centre for Health Policy and Evaluation. Her research interests include primary care, variations in practice patterns, the epidemiology of medical care, and assessment of the effectiveness and outcomes of medical interventions. Specific topics of interest focus on referral patterns and quality of care.

Allan Donner is Professor and Chairman, Department of Epidemiology and Biostatistics, University of Western Ontario. His major research interests focus on methodological issues that arise in epidemiology, health care research, and clinical trials. Recent examples include the development of methodology for clinical trials that randomize groups rather than individuals, the investigation of the robustness of standard statistical methods to violations of the assumption of statistical independence, and the development and evaluation of inference procedures for the analysis of family data. He did his undergraduate training at the University of Manitoba, where he also completed a master's degree. He received his doctorate from the Department of Statistics at Harvard University. He is currently President of the Biostatistics Section of the Statistical Society of Canada and on the Board of Editors of the *American Journal of Epidemiology*. In 1989, he was elected a Fellow of the American Statistical Association.

Earl V. Dunn has been Professor in the Department of Family and Community Medicine since 1982 and is also Professor at the Centre for Studies in Medical Education at the University of Toronto, Ontario, Canada. Born in the province of Quebec in 1931, he was educated in Quebec and New Brunswick and graduated from McGill University Medical School in 1960. He did a two-year general practice residency in Kansas City, Missouri, and then entered practice in a mining community in the Province of Quebec. In 1968, he became a full-time member of the Faculty of Medicine, University of Toronto. He has specific research interests in medical decision making, telemedicine, resource use, and the economics of health care delivery. He has also published in all these fields.

Robert H. Fletcher is Editor of the *Annals of Internal Medicine*, the official journal of the American College of Physicians. He was educated at Wesleyan University, Harvard Medical School, and

Johns Hopkins University School of Hygiene and Public Health. His clinical training was in internal medicine at Stanford and Johns Hopkins, where he was a fellow in the Clinical Scholars Program, a fellowship for research and policy training at the interface between clinical and population medicine, until becoming a full-time journal editor in 1990. He is an academic general internist and clinical epidemiologist. He began his faculty career at McGill University and moved to the University of North Carolina in 1978, where he was Director of the Robert Wood Johnson Clinical Scholars Program and Co-Director of the International Clinical Epidemiology Network training program. With his wife Suzanne Fletcher and colleague Edward Wagner, he wrote *Clinical Epidemiology: The Essentials*, a textbook that has been translated into six languages. More recently, he has been studying the effectiveness of peer review of manuscripts submitted for publication in medical journals.

Stephen H. Gehlbach is a pediatrician and epidemiologist by training but claims broad interest in health affairs, from promoting primary care research to reforming the U.S. health care industry. He is currently Dean of the School of Public Health at the University of Massachusetts, Amherst, where he occasionally clears his desk of administrative chores to teach courses in principles of epidemiology and communicable disease epidemiology. His research interests cover a broad range. He has worked in areas of agricultural occupational illness and poisoning, physician behavior change, and medical education. He is currently collaborating with a group at the University of Massachusetts, Amherst, who are developing models that estimate the probability of mortality among ICU patients.

Richard Glazier, MD, MPH, is Associate Professor at the University of Toronto in the Departments of Family and Community Medicine and Preventive Medicine and Biostatistics. He is based at the Wellesley Hospital, where he is a member of the hospital research institute's Division of Clinical Epidemiology. He is also a member of the Arthritis Community Research and Evaluation Unit, a health system-linked research unit based at the Wellesley Hospital, and an associate member of the University of Toronto's Centre for Health Promotion. He received his M.D. degree from the

University of Western Ontario and completed training in Family Medicine at Queen's University. After several years in family practice in Whitby, Ontario, he completed an M.P.H. degree and Preventive Medicine residency at Johns Hopkins School of Hygiene and Public Health. As part of his training, he spent one year in Geneva as a short-term consultant with WHO's Programme for Control of Acute Respiratory Infections. He is a certificant of the College of Family Physicians of Canada and board-certified by the American Board of Preventive Medicine. His current research projects include: (a) the epidemiology of childhood respiratory infections among aboriginal children in Northwestern Ontario; (b) the etiology of pneumonia among young infants at Toronto's Hospital for Sick Children; (c) psychosocial risk factors in pregnancy as related to screening tests and pregnancy outcomes; and (d) the role of the family physician in the delivery of care to people in Ontario with arthritis and related musculoskeletal disorders. He is active in teaching at the graduate level at the University of Toronto in Family Medicine, Clinical Epidemiology, and International Health.

Mary-Jo DelVecchio Good (Ph.D.) is Associate Professor of Medical Sociology, Department of Social Medicine, Harvard Medical School, and Associate Director of the Centre for the Study of Culture and Medicine at Harvard University. Her areas of research include the profession of medicine and cultural analyses of medical knowledge and medical practice. Her most recent publication is *Pain as Human Experience: An Anthropological Perspective* (University of California Press), which was written with P. Brodwin, B. Good, and A. Kleinman.

Brian K. Hennen, MD, is Chairman of the Department of Family Medicine at the University of Western Ontario. A medical graduate of Queen's University, he entered private practice in Orillia, Ontario. Returning to postgraduate clinical training in Pediatrics, Internal Medicine and Family Medicine, he completed an MA in Educational Psychology at Michigan State University and established a career in academic medicine at the University of Western Ontario. He served as Chairman of the Department of Family Medicine at Dalhousie University in Halifax, Nova Scotia, prior to his current appointment. He was the founding chairman of the section of Teachers of the College of Family Physicians of Canada and is a past president of that college. He is an Honorary Member of the Royal College of General Practitioners and a Fellow of the Westminster Institute of Ethics and Human Values.

Rebecca Henry is Associate Professor in the office of Medical Education Research and Development at Michigan State University in the College of Human Medicine. Her research interests include survey research methods, physician-patient communication skills, interventions to promote strategies of health promotion among primary care providers, and program evaluation. In 1991, she completed a sabbatical at the W. K. Kellogg Foundation conducting an evaluation of the Community Partnerships Program, a new initiative in health professions education. She is also interested in developing the research of physicians, residents, and medical students. She has numerous publications that focus on this topic and has collaborated on a book. She is frequently requested to present to different professional groups on how to develop research skills for the health professions.

Janis H. Jenkins is Assistant Professor of Anthropology at Case Western Reserve University. She received her doctoral training from the University of California, Los Angeles, and postdoctoral training at Harvard Medical School. As a psychiatric anthropologist, her research interests concern the course and outcome of major mental disorder, psychiatric disability among immigrants and refugees, and cultural analyses of psychiatric theory. She has worked extensively with Latin American and Latino populations in North America. Two recent publications include the 1990 Stirling Award essay: "Anthropology, Expressed Emotion, and Schizophrenia" (*Ethos, 19,* 1991) and a special article for the American Journal of Psychiatry titled "The Meaning of Expressed Emotion: Theoretical Issues Raised by Cross-Cultural Research" (*AJP, 149,* 1992). Currently, she is Principal Investigator for a 5-year study funded by the NIMH on psychocultural and socioenvironmental factors that may affect recovery from schizophrenia and depression.

Michel Labrecque is Assistant Professor in the Department of Family Medicine, Laval University, St. Foy, Quebec, Canada. His research interests are in evaluation of diagnostic and therapeutic interventions in primary care, mainly in the field of perinatal medicine and contraception, and in feasibility studies and evaluation of development programs in Third World countries.

Carol L. McWilliam is Assistant Professor jointly appointed to the Departments of Family Medicine and Nursing at the University of Western Ontario. She is the nurse-researcher of the Thames Valley Family Practice Research Unit, a multidisciplinary research partnership between the Centre for Studies in Family Medicine and the London Chapter of the College of Family Physicians of Ontario. Her research focuses on health services delivery, health promotion, and new applications of qualitative research methods. Specific projects include (a) a pilot study of the discharge experience of rural elderly patients sent home from a smaller acute care hospital with continued care needs; (b) a larger urban study to gain comparable understanding in that setting and to test the feasibility of using research assistants for qualitative health services research; (c) a community health promotion action research study of the process of addressing farmers' health concerns related to drinking water contamination; and (d) an intervention study to describe and test a health promotion process to assist elderly with chronic care needs to manage on their own at home. She also teaches research methodology and health care system issues, the former to both nursing and family medicine students and the latter in the Master of Science in Nursing program at the University of Western Ontario.

E. Ann Mohide is Associate Professor in the School of Nursing and the Department of Clinical Epidemiology and Biostatistics at McMaster University. She is also the Senior Nurse Researcher at the Hamilton Regional Cancer Centre and Director of the Supportive Cancer Care Research Unit, funded by the Ontario Ministry of Health, Health System-Linked Research Program. Her research includes community and institutionally based health services evaluation for chronic conditions.

Andrew D. Oxman graduated from medical school at Michigan State University in 1979. Following this, he lived in Norway for 5 years, where he undertook internship training and worked as a general practitioner in the north. He subsequently trained in Community Medicine at McMaster University. He is currently Assistant Professor at McMaster with a joint appointment in the Departments of Family Medicine and Clinical Epidemiology and Biostatistics. He has a cross appointment in the Hamilton-Wentworth Teaching Health Unit and a part-time attachment to the Health Information Research Unit. He is a Career Scientist of the Ontario Ministry of Health. The general focus of his research activities is on methods of improving the use of research evidence in clinical practice, public health, health behavior, and health policy.

Anthony J. Reid is currently Assistant Professor in the Department of Family and Community Medicine, Toronto General Hospital, part-time, as well as family physician in private practice in Orillia, Ontario. He received his M.D. at Toronto, his C.C.F.P. at Memorial University, and his M.Sc. in design, measurement and evaluation at McMaster University. His past experience includes family practice teaching units in St. John's and Toronto General Hospital as well as clinical practice in Northern Ontario, Malawi, East Africa, and Papua New Guinea. Research interests include obstetrics and family medicine, midwifery, and tropical health.

Leslie L. Roos graduated from Stanford University and received his doctoral degree in political science from the Massachusetts Institute of Technology. Before coming to the University of Manitoba in 1973, he held faculty positions at Brandeis, Northwestern, and Indiana universities. He has held a National Health Scientist Award from the Research Programs Directorate, Health and Welfare, Canada, since 1982. He is a member of the Department of Community Health Sciences (Faculty of Medicine) at the University of Manitoba. He is an Associate of the Canadian Institute for Advanced Research and Director of the Data Base at the Manitoba Centre for Health Policy and Evaluation.

Walter Rosser is Chairman of the Department of Family and Community Medicine at the University of Toronto. He formerly held the same position at McMaster University and the University of Ottawa. His main academic interests over the past 20 years have centered on the development of information systems for family practice offices and the use of these systems to study and attempt to improve prescribing and preventive activities in practice. More recently, he has been involved with guideline development and studies around changing physician behavior. He has a long-standing interest in the North American Primary Care Research Group and was a founding member of the Ambulatory Sentinel Practice Network. He is currently the president of both these organizations.

Milton H. Seifert, Jr., has been a family physician in full-time general practice in Excelsior, Minnesota, since 1961. He has academic appointments as Clinical Associate Professor, Department of Family Practice and Community Health, University of Minnesota, and Assistant Clinical Professor, Department of Family Medicine and Practice, University of Wisconsin. He and his associates have developed the Eagle Medical Model with the help of the Family Health Foundation of America, the Robert Wood Johnson Foundation, the Management Medicine Foundation, and a Small Business Innovative Research (SBIR) grant from the National Institutes of Health. He has served as the Chair of the Research Committee of the Minnesota Academy of Family Physicians from 1969 to 1989 and was named the 1990 Minnesota Family Physician of the Year. He is also a member of the Ambulatory Sentinel Practice Network, the Society of Teachers of Family Medicine, and the North American Primary Care Research Group. His primary interest is practice-based research.

Harvey A. Skinner (Ph.D.) is Professor and Chairman of the Department of Behavioral Science, Faculty of Medicine, University of Toronto. Also, he is a Senior Scientist at the Addiction Research Foundation, Toronto. He received his Ph.D. in psychology in 1975 from the University of Western Ontario and has been a Registered Psychologist in the Province of Ontario since 1976. He is a member of the Task Force on Curriculum Renewal in undergraduate medical education. During 1987-1990, he was a member of a study for the U.S. Congress on the Treatment of Alcohol Problems, conducted by the U.S. National Academy of Sciences. He has served as a Consulting Editor for both the *Journal of Abnormal Psychology* and the *Journal of Consulting and Clinical Psychology*. He was a member of the Board of Trustees, Toronto General Hospital, from 1982 to 1986. He was an adviser to a World Health Organization collaborating project on early intervention for alcohol problems and is an expert adviser to the U.S. National Institute on Alcohol Abuse and Alcoholism. He has been a pioneer in the use of microcomputer technology.

Sylvie J. Stachenko received her medical degree from McGill University in 1975. She completed her residency program in family medicine at the University of Montreal in 1975 and received a master's degree in epidemiology and in health services administration from the Harvard School of Public Health in 1985. She has been Associate Professor with the Department of Family Medicine at the University of Montreal since 1987. She has been involved with the development of family medicine research in Quebec as Director of Research in the Department of Family Medicine and as President of the Quebec Research Group in family medicine from 1985 to 1988. Her main research interests include evaluation of preventive strategies and health services research. In 1990, she was appointed Director of the Division of Prevention in the Department of National Health and Welfare and is responsible for the development of policies in chronic disease prevention in Canada. She is also the current Canadian Director for the WHO-CINDI international chronic disease prevention program.

Fred Tudiver is a family physician and Associate Professor in the Department of Family and Community Medicine, University of Toronto, Canada. Born in Quebec, he was educated in McGill and Memorial Universities, and the University of Western Ontario. He was in community practice in London, Ontario, 1975-1979, and has been in academic practice ever since, both at Memorial and the University of Toronto. His research interests include primary prevention, in particular with the use of mutual support; the development of survey instruments for primary care settings; primary care involvement with wife abuse; and the content and evaluation of psychotherapy by family physicians.

J. Ivan Williams is Deputy Director of the Clinical Epidemiology Unit at the Sunnybrook Health Science Centre. He is a Professor at the University of Toronto and holds academic appointments in the Department of Family and Community Medicine, the Department of Preventive Medicine and Biostatistics, and the Faculty of Nursing. His primary research interests are health care evaluation, assessing outcomes, and methods for measuring quality of life. His research projects include quality assessments in family medicine, the evaluation of prehospital emergency services, and related resource use, practice procedures, and outcomes.

Dennis G. Willms (Ph.D.) is Assistant Professor in the Department of Clinical Epidemiology and Biostatistics and an associate member in the Department of Anthropology at McMaster University, Hamilton, Ontario, Canada. He is also a faculty member for the International Clinical Epidemiology Network (INCLEN), a Rockefeller Foundation-funded training program for international scholars, and is Co-ordinator of the social science component in the McMaster University Training Unit. His research interests include the systematic use of qualitative and ethnographic research methods in addressing health care problems in clinical and community-based settings. At the current time, he is involved in research projects in AIDS prevention (Uganda and Zimbabwe) and supportive cancer care (Canada).

Douglas M. C. Wilson is Professor in the Department of Family Medicine, Faculty of Health Sciences, McMaster University. He has been an investigator or principal investigator on six clinical trials related to smoking cessation as well as principal investigator in studies of health maintenance, exercise prescribing, and chlamydia screening. He is currently an investigator on a multicenter community smoking intervention trial and is heading a College of Family Physicians' study on alcohol risk assessment and investigation. He has consulted on numerous projects related to health promotion, including the NIH/NCI Physician Intervention in Smoking Manuals and Teaching Packages; the American Academy of Family Physicians' Smoking Cessation Kit; the Canadian Council on Smoking and Health's Consensus Recommendations for Physician Interventions with Smokers; Crisco's Physician Recommendations for Dietary Assessment and Counselling; and Homewood Health Centre's Drinkwise Project. He also supervises family practice residents at the McMaster Medical Centre's Family Practice Clinic. He was the Medical Director of this clinic for 7 years and the Education Committee Chairman for the past 5 years.